Helichrysum: for The Wound That Will Not Heal:

The Lost History of Immortelle, The Everlasting Flower, Its Chemistry and Helichrysum Italicum Essential Oil Uses in Aromatherapy

Form Misty, because she is just beginning to understand there is so much more to an aromatherapy treatment than safety, dilution and blending.

With much love x

Knock, knock

Who's there?

Doctor...

Dr Who?

You just said it!

Introduction

Don't look for The Doctor. He's not here. For we are visiting a time lord of a different kind, an everlasting plant, the one they call immortelle or even the "unwithering one, the amaranth".

For the journey though, we require a time machine because frankly my legs aren't as good as they used to be and to discover the plant lost in history, then we do need to do quite a lot of nipping about.

We'll be traversing through time, zipping backwards and forth so ladies, grab your moisturisers please. A Helichrysum one will work decidedly well for this journey. The oil of regeneration seems just the thing, for time differences will give you nothing if not jet lag and wrinkles. It's best we go armed with protection.

I am pretty sure you don't need your passport to travel in a Tardis but I'm never sure how much to pack. Since we are heading off to Rome and Ancient Greece it might be worth changing the bed. I hear sheets are quite the thing. One just never knows what festivities one will get invited to, does one? I'd hate to see you underdressed. Oh and by the way you might want to grab yourself a bottle of rosehip carrier, just in case.

So why the Tardis and why Dr Who? Well, as you read the book you will come to a discover a plant that has always been revered because it is everlasting. More than that though, in more recent clinical trials we can see that it has a unique part to play in [cell] regeneration. It moves in an out of time in the strangest of fashions and very like the Tardis, it seemed to suddenly pop up out of no-where without explanation!

It was Kurt Schnaubelt who pointed the strange idiosyncrasy of the essential oil. That mentions of it could not found in any aromatherapy books before the 1980s but, still, it had been accepted into the therapist's box and indeed is probably the one of the most beloved of our oils. When there is very little historical evidence of usage by the ancients, how did that happen? Well, that is a very interesting question worth pondering, I felt.

I have always been interested in Helichrysum, mainly because actually I *wasn't* that interested in it and I seemed to be the only one! Everyone seemed to be lauding its graces and my bottle seemed to sit eternally happy at the back of the box, slowly collecting dust on the oily top! What was it about this mysterious oil that seemed the capture other healer's imagination so?

That makes it sound like I never use it. (I do; I just don't dust!!!) I have always used it for strengthening, as an overall tonic, and in more recent years have also used it for healing skin. I had heard it tell that the best scarring panacea grew in Corsica but I had no real understanding of why the difference might exist apart from obvious soil differences.

At Botanica 2016, I was signing books and sharing a stall with an oil's company called Sanatio Naturalis. We had been situated in a room full of the most amazing artisan distillers from Arizona, Greece, Syria and Iceland. It was like being in Heaven for an oil junkie like me. Opposite us was the very prettiest stand of Helichrysum oils and hydrolats, wild harvested from plants grown on a remote island just off the coast of Croatia. The golden yellow labels on the brown bottles were interspersed through glorious royal blue earthenware oil burners and pictures of the yellow Helichrysum growing against the blue sky of Croatia. I was bowled over. When I smelled their bottle of oil, I was utterly captivated. A whole new realm of consciousness seemed the rush in and I had to know more.

Back home, a great tragedy had touched my family's lives. My daughter's best friend had been involved in the most awful crash. She had been in a coma and had come out of it left with hideous brain injuries and skin grafts on her back, arms and hands that refused to stay closed. I felt compelled to learn more about the oil that I understood might be able to help the skin to heal. I believed this oil had much to give (Although remember the one that is good for is Corsican Helichrysum and I had fallen in love with the Croatian one but I wouldn't be told!)

So when I got home I started, as always, by looking on the internet. Most of the authorities seemed to agree there was little to draw from history, except for some scanty references by Dioscorides, Pliny and Theophastrus and some cultural significance delivered by Pliny.

This seems to be as good a place as anywhere to start, so climb into the Tardis, set the dial to AD70 and let's find out what they had to say.

PS: If you are a reader who only loves reading the clinical aspects of the oil, and does not like the metaphysical, I am going to ask you to close the preview now, and do not buy this book. You are not going to enjoy this particular one and I'd rather you saved your money. George Shepherd (Amazon) *has done a book with most of the same science as I have and, on this occasion, I am going to say buy his book instead. My book is seriously spooky and he and I end up in the same labs eventually. It saves me getting rubbish reviews. Thanks!*

Table of Contents

Introduction....................3

Table of Contents....................7

History....................11

Dreams....................22

The Sacred Flower of The Goddess....................23

The Festival- Amarysia....................26

Etymology....................29

Synonyms....................30

Amaranth The Everlasting....................31

The Funeral Wreath....................34

The Kama Sutra....................39

Helichrysum italicum (Roth) G.Don....................46

Botany....................46

Chemistry....................47

Chemotypes of Helichrysum italicum essential oil....................50

Corsican Helichrysum....................51

Tuscan Helichysum....................51

Croatian Helichrysum....................52

Sardinian Helichrysum....................53

Ethnobotany....................54

The Metaphysical Aspects of Helichrysum's Healing....................61

Archetype....................61

Medical Astrology of Chiron....................69

Medical Astrology of The Sun....................74

Helichrysum's Healing Journey Through Chiron....................74

Chiron in the natal chart....................98

Helichrysum Healing of the Physical Body with Aromatherapy 124
Skin 124
Scarring 124
Burns 127
Acne 127
Abscesses 127
Eczema, Dermatitis and Psoriasis 128
Anti-allergenic 128
Radiation burns 128
Inflammation 128
Blood 129
Bruises 130
Thrombosis 130
Phlebitis 131
Coronary complaints 131
Haemorrhoids 131
Varicose veins 131
Arterial Circulation (Hozzel) 131
Liver 131
Hepatitis 132
Digestive system 132
Respiratory 133
Genito Urinary 133
Reproductive 134
Hearing Problems 134
The Emotional Healing of Helichrysum 135
Magickal Uses: 138
Clinical Evidence of *Helichrysum italicum* 138

Using Helichrysum in your treatments 157
Blending 157
Safety Data 157
Undiluted Usage 157
Ingestion 158
Recommended Dilution 158
Drug Interactions 159
The Musical Vibration of Helichrysum 163
Conclusion 169
Learn from The Secret Healer 175
About The Author 175
Other Books by the Author 177
References 180
Disclaimer 192
Recipes 195
Skin Repair After Operation 195
Blood Thinning 195
Reduction of Cholesterol 195
Heart Protection 195
Liver Protection 196
Gall Bladder 196
Pancreas 196
Anti-Inflammatory 197
Chirotic Abscesses 197
Stretch Marks 197
Digestive 198
Coughs and Chest congestion 198
Anti-Aging Moisturiser 199

Toner 199
Acne treatment 199
Metaphysical 201

History

We'll start by listening to Dioscorides. He speaks of our plant in his *De Materia Medica.* It is a useful piece of source material because, not only is it a collection of around 600 plant synopses but it also elucidates earlier works that were written by Theophastrus. In other words, his work tends to fill in the gaps that history has lost from Theophastrus's.

So translated from the early Greek, the Dioscorides text we need to refer to is: 4-57.

Immediately you will notice that Helichrysum's name has changed a bit. Get used to that. It is going to happen a lot! The translator has kindly added in who classified and traced the plant lineage (Fuchs 16th Century and Linnaeus 18th Century)

It reads:

ELICHRUSON SUGGESTED:

Amarantus luteus, Stichas citrina, Helichryson [Fuchs], Gnaphalium arenarium [Linnaeus], Helichrysum arenarium [in Sprague], Helichrysum chinophylum, Helichrysum arenarium — Helichrysum, Cudweed, Eternal Flower, Golden Sunflower

He tells us:

Helichrysum (with which they crown their statues) has a little stem — white, green, straight and strong — and narrow leaves (similar to those of abrotanum) set apart at distances, the filaments circular, shining like gold; a round tuft, (as it were) dry bunches of berries, and a thin root. It grows in rough places near running water.

He describes the usage:

A decoction of the filaments (taken as a drink with wine) helps painful urination, the bites of snakes, sciatica, and hernia. A decoction (taken as a drink with must [pulp from grapes]) induces the menstrual flow, and dissolves clots of blood in the bladder or bowels. Thirty grains in a dilution of white wine (given to one fasting) stops dripping fluids. It is stored together with clothes, protecting them from moths. It is also called chrysanthemon, ***while some call it amarantum.***

Note the underline. This will become important.

So we know it has lots of names and that it was in usage in Dioscorides lifetime which is thought to be AD40-90. We also know it was in usage *where* he lived. He was a native of Cilicia, Asia Minor and spoke Greek. He worked as a surgeon in the Roman Army under Nero so this also gives us context. His travels would have taken him all over the Roman Empire, a very useful perk for someone who liked to study and collect native plants. More importantly for our research we now know he can speak for two civilisations, he understands what was happening in the Roman world of medicine but also the Greek. Likewise, because he was such an adept scholar, it is likely he would have been very interested in the medicines he came into contact with *during* his travels. One such civilisation was the Etruscans (known as Tyrrhenians by the Greeks).

The Etruscans and the Romans had had a long and unusual relationship. Originally *subjects* of the Etruscans who lived just north of Rome on the river Arno, the Romans eventually *overpowered* the nation. The nation's power had been at its greatest at around 1300BC and their wealth came from agriculture and mineral resources from their homeland which is what we would now call Tuscany. Eventually the Romans finally seized control in 296BC.

In an academic paper from 2010 we find evidence that the Etruscan civilisation used Helichrysum as one of their primary medicines. The study entitled "*Were natural forms of treatment for Fasciola hepatica available to the Etruscans?*" by Harrison et al. is very useful to us. Their research had been into the Etruscan practice of divination from sheep livers. This was a skill that the Romans were very impressed by and subsequently they also took up the practice. The study had highlighted that the liver could often be diseased. From this details then, they had wanted to identify if the Etruscans had known of any plants that might have been useful for treating *Fasciola hepatica* (Liver fluke) infection.

Their findings move us forward a great deal here. Based on their research from Dioscorides (833 Diosc. 4.58 RV) they had found out three things.

Firstly, that Etruscans had knowledge of Helichrysum and their name of the flower was **Garuleum**. That in Greece it could be called **Chrysanthemon** or **Chalkar.** The Latin was **Caltha** and the modern names are **Bronze Flower, Helichrysum and Immortelle.** I'm going to add **Everlasting Flower** to that list.

It would be useful, at this point to tell you the tiniest bit of taxonomy. The Helichrysum genera is big. What I mean by big, is *huge*. There are over 600 different species carrying the name Helichrysum. The plant most used in aromatherapy is *Helichrysum italicum (or Helichrysum angustifolium).* However, this plant genus is famed for being incredibly difficult to classify and so often there is mis-identification of the species. (Strangely, experiments now show that because the essential oil profiles are so different from place to place, it is currently thought the best way to identify the plant is by looking at the essential oil first so the chemistry now leads the classification!) Identification would have been incredibly difficult two millennia ago, as it is today, so although we are not going to cover 600 species, we will look at similar species to the *italicum* we have come to know and love. Here, for example we are moving a little bit away from the species he is talking about. Nevertheless, the data are useful.

The second thing the study tells us is: Immortelle - *Helichrysum arenarium* is **a member of the Daisy family**.

Lastly they tell us that Pliny the Elder, said in the first century, that **Immortelle was used for crowning the gods.** Pliny knows this from Theocrites who tells that it was used during the Ptolemy dynasty (Egypt; 330-305 B.C.): 'the plant comes from the metamorphosis of a nymph and is used for **making crowns and garlands'.** (*Lynda Farrar tells us this nymph was the first to pick the bloom and her name was Helichryse.)*

Dioscorides mentions another species, *Helichrysum sanguineum*, and explains that this, too, "*is like 'bākkaris', with aspect of grass and with rough leaves **it is used to make crowns**.*"

Pliny refers to these statements in his book XXIX. He comments: "of Heliocriso there refers Dioscorides (4.57), the yellow everlasting (helikhryson). Golden flower (khrysanthemon) **and a different** that does not withered (amaranths). With this one the images are crowned also".

So what is he saying? That there are two?

Yes, it is. There are two types of amaranth used to crown idols. One is golden and another is purple.

In the book XXI (47) Pliny tells us: *Amaranto not dubie vincimur. Spica is autem purpurea Verius flos quam aliquis ... postquam defecere cuncti flores, madefactus aqua revivescit and hibernae coronas facit* .

Translation: We certainly cannot compete with amaranth. This is indeed a purple spike rather than a flower ... when all the flowers have gone, she comes alive when quenched in water, and is used to make winter wreaths.

Later, he tells us it is a purple stem again but then adds it has morc than onc flowcr and is itsclf odourless". Here he speaks about the Amaranth we still know today: Celosia argentea. That it has no scent will become useful to know later.

Dioscorides agrees and in IV (58) he demonstrates: "The Elicriso called by a few Chrysanthemom (Chrysanthemum) and by other Amaranton (Amaranthus), it is a certain plant which is usually crowned the idols. Called also amaranth because their flowers last infinitely without corruption and without loses smell, which indicates this name amaranth. **There are two species of ordinary amaranth: the yellow one**, which the barbarians call 'sticados citrina' and another purple so called 'flower amoris' or flower of the love.

Barbarians is a term much changéd through history. At the point of Dioscoride's writing it would have been used to denote anyone who did not speak Greek. Later the Visigoths took on the mantle when they broke down the Roman Empire. From then, the term morphed into a word used to describe evil people performing dreadful acts. Hence at the time of writing no evil is implied by the fact these Non-Grecians gave his precious plant a different name!

To summarise then, both authorities tell us there are two separate species that do not wither; one is of the family ***Asteraceae*** and other one of ***Amaranthaceae*** and they were used to crown the gods, idols and the dead.

The descriptions from Pliny and Dioscorides agree in identifying Helichrysum, most likely they are referring to H. sanguineum which they both list between plants that are sedative, hypnotic, psychotropic or narcotic. Pliny explains he is citing Egyptian wisdom here: "*Helicriso, flower that it does not withered, called immortal, which crowned their gods, as says Ptolemy, king of Egypt. This plant believed that it contributed to the fame and glory who was crowned with her the three Wise Men too. It is a flower like gold, which garlands and ointments give benevolence and glory, stored in golden glasses that call apiron*".

Could our plant have been the source of the powers of the three wise men? I find no other references to this.

In 'Historia Naturalis' XXI *Pliny further writes "Eliocriso, some call as chrysanthemum: it have white stems, whitish leaves seemed to the 'abrotino'* (Abrotino is Santolina-Asteraceae), *when it reached for the Sun 15 comes shine as gold and they never fade. For this reason, the gods are crowned, and protecting the clothes with his smell*".

Later in the same work Pliny regales many different plants that can be found in unguents and ointments of the period. The list is extensive and whilst it does not point directly to Helichrysum, he does mention *abrotino* and says that the two can often be confused.

Right. Time to jump in the blue telephone box....

Set it to 300 years further in the past please.

Theophrastus preceded Dioscorides by around about three centuries. Although he did not mention this plant *Amaranthus* directly, he wrote with a good degree of scepticism about the "magical properties" of a "gold-flower" of which Pliny had raved so eloquently.

Get ready, he gets most irate!

So too what is said of good or fair fame as affected by plants is quite as foolish or more so: for they say that the plant called snapdragon produces fair fame. This plant is like bedstraw but it has no root: and the fruit has what resembles a calf's nostrils.

The man who anoints himself with this they say wins fair fame. And they say that the same result follows, if he crowns himself with the flower of gold-flower, sprinkling it with unguent from a vessel of unfired gold. The flower of gold-flower is like gold, the leaf is white. The stem also is white and hard, the root is slender and does not run deep.

Men use it in wine against the bites of serpents, and to make a plaster for burns after burning it and mixing the ashes with honey. Such tales then, as was said before, proceed from men who desire to glorify their own crafts

The properties he recites are very similar to those Dioscorides cites. The botanical description fits. But we have a different slant here because most of what we have read seems to suggest that the wreaths are put onto statues but that's not what he is saying is it? He's scoffing that many people believe that if they use the macerated oil of the gold flower onto their bodies it will imbue them with some kind of power. Further he suggests people who sell it are charlatans only looking to make a quick buck with these claims. (Not much changes, does it?)

But not everyone feels the same way. In the 3rd century AD, Athenaeus of Naucratis refutes Theophastrus's assertion in his work the *Deipnosophistae. (The Deipnosophistae* is a bit of an unusual work. In many ways, one could suggest it is little more than ramblings of learned people at the dinner table after rather a few too many glasses of vino. It draws on factoids and fables from any number if subjects, philosophy, history, cookery. Not least it speaks in detail of magical spells that Atheneaus assures us, in Grecian life, count in the many. It is thought to be the world's oldest surviving cookbook. It is within this strange set of information that Athenaeus argues his point saying Theophastrus is mistaken and that the plant is indeed magical and capable of great things.

Wait a minute though. We have skipped away from something interesting I think. Theophastrus mentions an unguent. So what unguent? What unfired gold vessel? I hear you plead.

I only wish I knew.

Pliny mentioned them too, didn't he? He mentions golden vessels called Apirons. I cannot find any more information on these.

It seems like they may have been something similar to this *Bakkaris* that Dioscorides spoke of or perhaps *brenthon* or *brentheion Myron*. These are names of cosmetics cited throughout Greek and Roman literature. Bakkaris (bakcharis, baccar), though, is more fully documented than the others. It is described by Greek writers of the mid-seventh right through to the fifth centuries BC. The earliest of these came from two Ionian poets, Semonides of Amorgos and Hipponax of Ephesus. Both of these originally hailed from places close to an area called Lydia and were contemporaries to the last of Lydian kings. For this reason, we refer to these unguents as *Lydian cosmetics.*

As ever, there is confusion as to whether the Bakkari were the plants they were made from or the actual unguent itself. It's likely it was both. (This feels like déja vu of Nard in my spikenard book.) We are not sure whether it was a dry powder, or a liquid, again it seems like it may have been both. Suggested plant sources of the Bakkarris are fox gloves, or *Helichrysum sanguineum* which has red flowers. Now that would be interesting, wouldn't it? Try to visualise if we could think of the redness of our more modern red unguent, Sea Buckthorn, being poured over yellow flowers. It would indeed shine like burnished gold! Add to that, archeological evidence shows that later Greeks began to add copper leaves into their Helichrysum wreaths and head dresses and we have a rather extraordinary sight beginning to form.

Interestingly it also seems that these bakkarris did indeed have their own types of container, which looked like Grecian vases, called Lydions. Perhaps these are the apirons we were looking for. I cannot tell.

Dreams

In III (46), Dioscorides describes that Helichrysum's smell **causes dreams** and that is re-iterated by our next Tardis stop. We are going *Back to The Future*, Marty (oh c'mon you knew that had to happen somewhere!!!) to the second century AD. I'm taking you to meet my mate Artemidorus. Now he's a very interesting fellow, so grab yourself a glass of wine and come over and see what he has to say.

He's a professional diviner, you know. *Interprets* dreams, no less. He has written five books on the subject. The first three are for laypeople like you and I, who are interested in the stuff of dreams; but the last two are for his son's eyes only, novice dream interpreter, as he is. Artemidorus comes from impressive stock, *eighteenth* in a long line of diviners! What he has to say is very interesting (reader, these books are still in existence today) because they say very similar to what Jung re-asserted two thousand years later. Namely, that dreams are symbols of one's reality.

Collected from many years of travelling around Greece, gathering testimony of other diviners, he tells us that the Greeks and Romans **would hang wreaths of amaranth in the temples of their most loved deities**. That its **themes**

are of strength and being immortal. He explains that **wreaths of amaranth will help anyone to reach success**, because, all year round, the amaranth keeps its fresh colour. The flower indicates strength and power.

It imbues strength to fight our fears.

Does it now Artemidorus? That is very interesting.

In his work *Interpretation of Dreams* he went on to explain that to **dream of wearing such a wreath of amaranth is good luck if one is in good health**. It is **especially lucky if one is going to court**, because the amarant keeps its colour, but it is **bad luck for the sick as these flowers are dedicated to the dead or to the gods and only rarely are they given to (living) people.**

Rarely given to living people....

Well that's weird isn't it?

Perhaps not. Because if you look up the term amaranthus, it gives a rather extraordinary explanation.

"*Amaranthus- meaning sacred to Artemis*".

The Sacred Flower of The Goddess

Having the name Amaranth means our Helichrysum was consecrated to the ancient hunter goddess Artemis. Legend has it that Amarynthus was a hunter and a son of the king of Euboea who came from a village also called Amarynthus. He was the lover of Artemis and often they would hunt together in the woods. One day it is said he made a snarky remark about Neptune, and Poseidon sent a wave to wash over him and drowned him. Then Artemis changed his body into an amaranth, because it was an everlasting flower.

So who was Artemis?

She was a very ancient goddess whose myths probably far predate the Ancient Greek civilization. They whisper of ancient religions far before patriarchal tones were overlaid upon her story.

Importantly she was a virgin goddess. The meaning of that is somewhat dissimilar to how we would conceive it today. It would need to be. She took Amarantus as her lover. In this context it means that she did not require a man to complete her. She had asked her father Zeus to grant her eternal chastity and virginity, and thus she rejected marriage and love devoting her life to hunting and nature. She is a well formed individual who never needed to marry to make her tale.

She is a huntress and may have been formed from the far more ancient goddess, Selene, of the moon. She was the goddess of chastity, virginity, the hunt, the moon, and the natural environment. She hunts at night and is fiercely protective of her clan. She was born of Leto, in a very easy birthing, but she was one of twins, her brother being Apollo. She is reputed to have dragged her mother to safety on an island and helped to birth her brother. For this reason, as she does not have children of her own she is seen as the protector of midwives.

She represents the feminine archetype of nature and the wilderness. The function of virgins was to dispense the Mother's grace to heal. They prophesied, performed sacred dances, and they wailed for the dead.

If you see statues of her, despite not having children of her own, she is seen with many breasts all over her torso. conveying her as the fertile nurturer of all living things. She was a huntress, a spectacular archer and a brilliant plant healer. Paradoxically the huntress was the killer/destroyer of the very creatures she had nurtured and helped to birth. Here we see the light and dark side of the goddess.

She dwelt in the forest and only came out at night. For this reason, she was to be called "the seeker of light". There is a real wrath in Artemis. We see her reeking absolute vengeance on several parties including Actaeon who had stumbled across her bathing in the forest, unable to look away when she asked him to, she turned him into a stag and then he was ripped to pieces by his own hunting hounds. Orion too, befell her wrath, albeit by accident when Apollo had told Artemis that one of her hand maidens had been raped. Apollo pointed out a speck in the distance (knowing very well it was Orion) and Artemis shot him.

She is a gentle but vengeful goddess and as such she exposes and embraces the dark side of the psyche.

Artemis was a very celebrated goddess who was revered for many centuries across many geographic areas. Her temples were spectacular. Many of us will have heard of the Temple of Artemis at Ephesus. In these temples, were held magnificent festivals called the *Amaranthia,* in praise and worship of Artemis. The first of these was held at the famous temple of Artemis Amarynthia, and then later moved to Attica where the name of the festival was also changed to Amarysia.

The Festival- Amarysia

The cult of Amaranthus was a very important sect of Amyrisia. They held the greatest of Artemis's annual festivals, the Artemiria.

Do you want to go? We've got the blue box if you fancy it. To my mind it seems a bit scary.

It seems that dramas playing out the kouretic myths were a major feature of these rites. The principal cult centre seems to have been situated in Amarynthis which the first century writer Strabo explains was "*seven staeds from Eritria*". The festival was celebrated at Anthestiron (that's in March to you and I) as Earth began to waken from her slumber.

Much of our knowledge of the festival comes from the Great Decree, IG XII. A large Roman inscription, the decree tells the story of a Macedonian officer at war with Athens. Written from a male civilian's point of view we are able to get a very good idea of the contests and rules of the festival.

The writer speaks in detail about sacrifices made. We know that these took place over a five day period and their nature reveals a great deal about the goddess. The decree tells us that there were to be sheep and bulls sacrificed and it is made clear that these are specifically "Selected". Now, this is unusual, because whilst most Olympian gods were believed to feast on oxen, sacrifices of sheep were rare. Moreover, traditional sacrifice etiquette meant you picked your strongest, fittest and most deserving specimen in a bid to please the gods. It should not be defective in any way. Artemis however, demanded that the sacrifices were to be of maimed or defective sheep.

The decree tells us that before the feasting began there was an inspection of the sacrificial animals and also a discussion about reimbursement of costs for the supervisors of the animals.

There was a fair, a carnival, a market, probably of food but perhaps candles, flowers and trinkets too.

Then was the gathering of the procession of those who wished to sacrifice, first the public officials with their offerings followed by the commoners.

There was an edict given that behaviour must be befitting for the occasion and then a magnificent band of chariots, military and hoplites processed behind. (Hoplites: If that's a new term to you, think Greek Soldier, leather tunic, helmet and spear!)

Rather than being true military, it has been suggested these were aristocratic demonstrations of status, that happened annually, regardless of whether the tribe was at war or not. A fairly late Grecian urn was found close to the area, depicting a warrior on a chariot which leads to the suggestion that these festivities, may have even continued regularly as late as the 6th century

Before the festival reached its climax, a spectacular dramatic ballet took place, the pyrrhic dance. Performed by fresh faced sixteen to nineteen-year-old military trainees, this leaping spectacle has many versions throughout history, often dedicated to Mars or other war deities. With a fast paced meter, the footwork demonstrates the lightning speed required to avoid spears and arrows. Many of the ancient poets describe how the crowds roared as the troupes entered the stadia, dancing their most beloved phyrric dance.

Traditional Greek Pyrrhic Dance: https://www.youtube.com/watch?v=cYelSpTWVUw

Close your eyes, hear the music, imagine the air rich with the fragrance of the thousands of garlands of helichrysm dedicated to the goddess, the frenzy of the crowds as their nubile young warriors entered the city walls and headed for the temple where they were to witness the sheep sacrifice.

But why were the young men there at all? It seems likely this was some sort of initiation ceremony for them, into the military or otherwise. They were brought here in the bid that Artemis would guard and protect them in her ministry.

Bear in mind, in the same way that in the Rose book we saw that Inanna, Venus, Isis etc were all representations of procreation, fertility and war, this also stands true for Artemis too, so therefore I suppose this could also be their way of blessing the crops. This would stand especially true I suppose for the purple amaranth in particular, because it its grain is such a valuable food source. A bitter trade.

A sacrifice of a different type. For fertile crops we offer you our young men to be sent into battle.

Etymology

Right, I think the safest place for the Tardis to go now is to the British Library because we need to go there later, and they should have some good dictionaries. Looking at the etymology, for a moment, helps us gain a deeper understanding of the symbolism surrounding the plant.

The Latin name was initially borrowed from the Greek. Ἀμάραντον – ***amaranton***.

This word appears in Dioscorides used as a synonym for χρυσοκόμη - ***khrusokomê*** (4, 55). Later studies by linguistics scholars have pinpointed this as *Aster linosyris* or ἑλίχρυσον - helikhruson and as such then identified as *Eastern Helichrysum* , *Helichrysum stoechas* or *Helichrysum sicelum* .

Synonyms

In popular literature, you might also see immortelle referred to as everlasting flower, St. John's weed (don't confuse it with St John's wort which is hypericum) yellow chaste weed, Italian straw flower, Herbe de St. Jean, immortel, and of course curry plant because the leaves smell like curry when they are crushed. (Although it is not the herb that is used to make masala curry powder.)

The difference between *H. angustifolium* and *H. italicum* are the same plant simply different names, according to Ernest Guenther (1948).

Often throughout this book though we refer to *H. stoechas,* which is a distinct variety, and when *H. angustifolium* and *H. stoechas* are distilled together, this is referred to as "oil of Helichrysum." Do not confuse this with Helichrysum essential oil, which should be italicum.

Clearly the name Helichrysum means something akin to "Golden Sun" in Greek, or perhaps it is thought, turning, sun.

The ancient name αμαραντος (never withering, literally "immortelle"), gestures to the legendary stamina it lends in times of environmental hardship. It is not a fussy plant. It can grow in very harsh terrains and can often be found growing out of a rocky outcrop.
Greek names:

amarantos, the unfading,

helikhryson, turning gold

khrysokomê, the golden-haired.
In France they call it simply "Petit soleil", little Sun.

The Spaniards refer to it as "scoba bedionda" meaning "smelly broom" a description of its to the strong and heavy fragrance.

In Belgium and in the Netherlands, they refer to Helichrysum as "*Strobloem*" because the flowers wither slowly.

Amaranth The Everlasting

The term *amaranth*, at the turn of the First Millennium had many connotations from its meaning. Not only was it botanical or even *ethno*botanical but it also came to have religious, literary and philosophical ramifications too.

Helichrysum = Amaranth = Everlasting

Originally the word is a verb derived from

μαραίνω - marainô ,

this means "to die, or to fade". Within the literal meaning it translates to a plant "that does not wither" or "never dies". Its exact equivalent is the French word for "immortal". This term was particularly used for plants used to make wreaths.

A good demonstration of usage is found in the Greek New Testament, 1 Peter 5:4,

"ton amarantinon tes doxes stephanon"

("the unfading crown of glory") *(And when the Chief Shepherd appears, you will receive the crown of glory that will never fade away*) and also in 1 Peter 1:4,

"kai amaranton" ("will not fade away") (*and into an inheritance that will not fade away. This inheritance is kept in heaven for you)*

Whilst scholars have not commented on this, I find it interesting that this also seems to purport to be some kind of bonus or award or specifically in 5:4 a wreath or crown.

Centuries later herbalists of the period followed Dioscoride's lead of there being two amaranth and transferred all of the associations from "helichruson" to the amaranth. In his 1539 work *Medicinae Herbariae*, Joannes Ammonius Agricola refers to the amaranth as "flos honoris" alluding to the plant's capability to "bring honour"

Working back two hundred years, to the 13th century, the name became an attribute of the Virgin Mary, a symbol of immaculate immortality: "Amaranthus flos, sacro, qui non marcet, honore vigens" (Johanes Germanus 1460 in Marraccio 1693). You can see this symbolism in a painting by Botticini. Amaranth plants grow from the ruins of the palace of David where Madonna adores the sacred child (D'Ancona 1977).

More modern associations with the everlasting still exist. In Southern Europe, amaranth was used to decorate churches on Ascension Day (Skinner 1925; Cole 1979), Swiss peasant families also hang wreaths of it over their door on that day.

Pilgrims to the men-only monastery island of Mount Athos take bouquets of Helichrysum as a symbol of the life everlasting.

The Funeral Wreath

We have overwhelming documentary evidence, then, that this amarantus was used for wreaths for the dead and for the gods. Isn't a shame, we can't see what they were like?

Well actually we can.

Because this is the everlasting flower.

One was found at Hawara in Egypt when Flinders Petrie excavated the Roman necropolis. There he found many mummies with the most amazing portraits painted over their faces and amongst the goods buried with them. Oone of these Helichrysum wreaths which can now be found in the British Museum. There is still debate as to exactly which Helichrysum it is. Some say *Helichrsysum conglobulatum* whereas others say *stoechas.*

You will be short changing yourself if you do not hop over to the link below to see a picture of the wreath. It dates from the second or third century. Eighteen hundred years later...it looks immaculate. Sadly, I have not been able to identify whose tomb it was found in. You can see it here:

http://www.britishmuseum.org/research/collection_online/collection_object_details.aspx?objectId=465854&partId=1

In his report about the excavation entitled Hawara, Biahmu, and Arsinoe he described his findings about the wreaths that had been found with these beautiful mummies.

Of the plants which were introduced into, and cultivated in, Egypt, for the beauty of their flowers or for their aromatic odour, the following are represented in this collection: (1) the Lychnis cali- rosa, L. ; (2) the myrtle (Myrtus communis, L.) ; (3) a species of Immortelle (Gnaphalium luteo-album, L.) ; (4) the woody nightshade (Solatium dulcamara, L.); (5) the sweet marjoram (Origanum iMajorana, L.) ; (6) the Celosia argentca, L. ; (7) the bay laurel (Laurus nobilis, L.) ; and (8) the polyanthus narcissus (Narcissus Tazetta, L.).

Gnaphalium luteo-album, L is synonym for Helichrysum. Did you note too, that he has also found Celosia there? The two amaranths! Later he explains:

Wreaths on the heads, pectoral garlands, and staves of flowers bound together, are found in coffins of this age; the flowers are usually red roses or immortelles.

It seems likely that the Helichrysum was imported from Italy or Greece. Later these wreaths were made in a new way, incorporating more of the beautiful plants that are being seen imported into the area. Then we start to see Jasmine sambac,

Rosa ricardii, Indian lotus and marjoram flowers being added in and it is about this time that we also find they have added the copper leaves that I spoke of earlier.

So we know it was used in burials in the Roman era. Potentially that wisdom was then lost (and how that happened I'll address later) but I want to show you something rather exciting and unsettling. Helichrysum is being investigated as a pollen found on a very important piece of linen.

No less than the Turin Shroud.

The shroud was dismissed as a medieval fake when it was carbon dated in the 1980s. Recent advances in archeological technology have exposed this method of dating as being fallible in some cases and indeed there are teams in Italy who suggest this may be the case with the Turin Shroud. They, for example, have suggested the possibility that an earthquake in AD33 may have skewed the carbon dating because its enormity – 8.2 on the Richter Scale – could have released neutron particles from crushed rock which could make an x-ray like imprint on the cloth. Last year scientists at the University of Padua, in Northern Italy dated it to between 300BC and AD400 – still hundreds of years after Christ, who is believed to have died between 30-36AD.

Dr Maria Boi is a palynological expert from the University of the Balearic Islands. She investigates pollens in live and fossilised forms. On visiting the shroud in the museum in Turin, she realised that there had not been rigorous enough testing into the pollens on the linen and so this threw the conclusions that had been made about the dating into doubt. She obtained previously released microscope slides of the pollens and compared them with her extensive research into plants used in funeral rites and their uses.

Originally the slides had been used to try to get a picture of where the shroud had been and to plot its historical journey. However, Boi felt they could be used to show when it had originated. For the main part she found that the identifications of the team were correct except that one pollen had been misidentified. What had been previously been listed as *Gundelia* was, in fact, a plant she was very familiar with. It was Helichrysum pollen which would place the shroud, indeed as Mediterranean in origin.

The pollens had found their way onto the fabric fibres because they had been used in embalming oils. She tells us that the fabric is entirely covered in these tiny organisms and thus it seems likely that the body has been washed using an oil containing Helichrysum and several other plants which are more expected for the time and most of which you should now be able to guess, frankincense, myrrh, galbanum etc etc.

This discovery of Helichrysum is important because the information regarding ancient burials was not uncovered until the 17th and 18th centuries and so a medieval forger is unlikely to have known how to create an embalming oil. This then, asserts Boi, suggests the Shroud is not medieval, it belonged to a Jewish person (because many of the other pollens found adhere to the Jewish traditions found in Exodus and described in my Spikenard book) and was prepared in Asia Minor (already established and agreed by scholars) for a Roman burial. In addition it should be stated that through her work through Dioscorides and Pliny she feels the plant would not have been used for just any person. Helichrysum was used for crowning the heads of gods. If you take a look at pictures of the Shroud, then, I'm not sure about you, but that could be a crown of Helichrysum....

She suggests that further work now needs to be done on the slides because previously the focus was in trying to ascertain the geographical journey the Shroud had taken through the pollens but now with this new discovery and understanding into embalming oils it makes it easier to try to pinpoint its place in time too. She adds there are another 103 pollen species on the linen that have not yet been identified.

As an interesting aside, I found some research that some marigold species had been identified in plant remains preserved by the eruption of Vesuvius. I scoured every avenue to see if we could see Helichrysum there and I found reference to a house at Pompeii called The House of Amaranthus. It had been called this because the ancient sign was still preserved on the wall and so this was its original name. Inside seems to have been a bar, but also it looked like the person who lived there may have made wreaths because many were found there. I was not able to ascertain what flowers these were made of, however.

The poets of long ago also have several places where they speak of the amaranthus in funerals but especially in the case of Achilles. The great warrior who gave his name to our lovely yarrow plant has many versions written about his demise, but there seems to be a common understanding that amaranth played an important part. Homer describes the Thessalians as wearing crowns to Achilles funeral. Elsewhere he suggests Thessalus decorated Achilles's tomb with them. (The Oracle of Dodona had ordered that the tomb be visited on the anniversary of his funeral so this may not have been at the funeral but maybe some time later, either way he used amaranth). Elsewhere it is told that amaranth was scattered on his grave by the Thessallians.

Who were the Thessallians then? I wanted to know. Very hard to tell. Thessaly seemed to have been inhabited by many different tribes that had come from the North East. In *Religion and Society in Ancient Thessaly* by Maria Mili there is a list of the people who make up the area. She cites Pelasgians,

Lapiths, Perrhabians, Aibians, Magnesian, Myrmidians, Dorians and Biotions.

There are two things familiar to me in that list. The first is Lapiths. These were the people who were reputed to have had the fiercest battles with the centaurs. The centaurs were a mythical race half men, half horses. They were first spawned by the cloud-nymph Nephele after she was violated by the impious Lapith king Ixion. The next is Magnesian. Some sources have Nephele as being a Magnesian mare – hence why they were half human, half horse. Finally, Thessaly is where Saturn violated Philydra and the Centaur Chiron was conceived. The Thessalonian forests are where the Centaurs lived!

Could it be that the Helichrysum was scattered by Centaurs....?

Surely that doesn't make sense?

Hold that thought. We'll come back to that later.

Ok, so we could do with leaving the ancient Greeks for a while and we need to journey to around the Third Century, but this time we are journeying to India.

The Kama Sutra

Helichrysum, the amaranth, can also be found in the beguiling third century work, The Kama Sutra. Here too, we see mention of the plant, in vaguely medicinal terms but more as a plant with great reverence placed upon it. Scholars suggest that, whilst this may be Helichrysum there is, however, also a yellow version of the red amaranth.

It reads:

"On the manner of living of a virtuous women and of her behaviour during the absence of her husband. A virtuous woman... should keep the whole house well cleaned, and arrange flowers of various kinds in different parts of it, and make the floor smooth and polished so as to give the whole a neat and becoming appearance. She should surround the house with a garden, and place ready in it all the materials required for the morning, noon and evening sacrifices... In the garden she should plant beds of green vegetables, bunches of the sugar cane, and clumps of the fig tree, the mustard plant, the parsley plant, the fennel plant, and the xanthochymus pictorius. Clusters of various flowers such as the trapa bispinosa, the jasmine, the jasminum grandiflorum, the yellow amaranth, the wild jasmine, the tabernamontana coronaria, the nadyaworta, the china rose and others, should likewise be planted, together with the fragrant grass andropogon schaenanthus, and the fragrant root of the plant andropogon miricatus. She should also have seats and arbours made in the garden, in the middle of which a well, tank, or pool should be dug."

Looking at the list it is hard to discern which, in fact it might be. *Andropogon schaenanthus,* Camel grass we met in the spikenard book and, as the passage says, it is fragrant. There are several different species of jasmine and also he suggests *Tabernamontana coronaria*, another jasmine, all of which are fragrant. Our Helichrysum is fragrant, whereas the yellow amaranthus is not. I think that probably justifies the traditional thinking that this is our plant.

So why should our virtuous lady be plating these wonders and digging great big ponds? Well, recipes later throw light on how she should use her flowers.

Firstly, it appears in the section of recipes designed to enlarge the lingham...
"The same effect is produced if a man has connection with a woman who has bathed in the buttermilk of a she-buffalo mixed with the powders of the gopalika plant, the banu-padika plant and the yellow amaranth. "

Before you look girls, no, Amazon don't do She-Buffalo milk . I already checked. But also:

"The juice of the roots of the madayantaka plant, the yellow amaranth, the anjanika plant, the clitoria ternateea, and the shlakshnaparin plant, used as a lotion, will make the hair grow."

Yes, ladies and gentlemen, there is indeed a plant called *Clitoria ternateea*, extremely pretty, with rather obscene looking blue flowers. Someone else thought fit to rename it "pigeon wings" but I rather like Vātsyāyana version better. I am interested to know though...which hair are we talking about here? I'm not eager to be sporting the wild woman of Borneo look! Surely that makes it incredibly difficult to walk?

So what are we seeing here? A recipe or spell that will make a wife patiently faithful whilst her husband away, a suggestion that his erection will be bigger and stronger and also the suggestion that Helichrysum can help the hair grow.

Can it?

Wait and see....

The history fizzles out now. This is where we lose the trail of the amaranth unless you trace the actual word. It gets changed and morphed through time and becomes a religious synonym for things that are immortal or everlasting. The word seems to leave the plant behind so to speak.

By the second century, the rise of Christianity had meant that crowns had taken on a new weight. It was felt that wearing them was a pagan practice and was insulting to the memory of the crown of thorns.

Wreaths had been worn for almost a thousand years at festivals and religious ceremonies. They had been worn by the victors of the Games. They had come to be symbols of civic officials, and of Achilles and his conquering heroes. It was a distinguishing mark of a Christian that they chose *not* to wear a wreath.

This decision to refrain from wearing is mentioned by three prominent writers of the period. Tertullian mentions it in his work *De corona* and Clement of Alexandria defines the reasons in his *Paedagogos*. Both works are for Christians outlining rules and regulations for their acceptable ways of living. Tertullian emphasises that the wearing of a crown is a breach of loyalty to Christ. Clement is concerned, more, that a crown is exalting the wearer to a height of luxury that they should not entitle themselves to. That a crown is not useful makes it excessive and that wearer should aim for self-control and moderations in their behaviour. He explains Christians should enjoy life "temperately, as in Paradise" (*Paedagogos* 2. 8.71); those who seek the truth, should not "wear laurel leaves and fillets of wool and purple, but crowns of righteousness and leaves of self-control" (*Exhortation to the Greeks* (1. 9 P, Loeb 26). Minucius Felix defends the abstention from wearing crowns, probably to a pagan audience, by explaining that Christians are being respectful and considerate by separating themselves from pagan practices.

So the crowns were laid down and with them the weight of symbolism was lost for our Sun gold plant. It drifted away into the mists of time until it was needed again by a strange tribe of people called aromatherapists.

In Aromatica, Peter Holmes tells us that it was used in renaissance medicine for liver, gall bladder and respiratory complaint. I have found it in a couple of herbals, for example in John Parkinson's *Theatre of Plants* where he seems to chuckle that ladies call it Everlasting Golden Flower, but I did not find a great deal of information from that period.

Holmes then explains that it began to "rise Phoenix-like from the ashes of herbal medicine", when in the 1960's Helichrysum has its first documented steam distillation in France and was subject to scientific scrutiny. In 1978 Brian Lawrence reported that Helichrysum oils and absolutes were appearing on the market and by the 1980s everyone was talking about the essential oil dubbed "the Super arnica of Aromatherapy"

Helichrysum italicum (Roth) G.Don

Botany

Genus:

Asteraceae (Compositae) family

You might see this also listed as ***strawflower*** but this is a different plant. Formerly classified as a Helichrysum this has now been renamed *Xerochrysum bracteatum.*

Helichrysum italicum is a perennial member of the daisy family. Originally derived from Italy and the Balkan coastal regions of Adriatic. Somehow, at some point in history it found its way to Corsica where the climate is similar and the soil, also rich in silica, gave it the optimum conditions to thrive. So much so, that Helichrysum is gives Corsica its characteristic fragrance.

The essential oil of *Helichrysum italicum* is most concentrated in the flowering tops between the months of June and July (although second harvesting and distillations usually happen later in the year). Even then the oil content is very low. In many cases, it is as low as 1% yield from the plant matter. (I wonder if it is this lack of grease is the reason that they last so long?)

The oil is typically steam distilled from those famous yellow flowers.

The colour of the oil varies tremendously based on where the plant grew and the soil composition of the area. Oil which comes from Corsica or from the Balkan states is usually yellowy orange, in Croatia it has a rich deeper almost rusty hue. I have read that the oil from the French Alps is bluey green but this, I have not seen for myself.

The low yield is only one contributing factor as to why Helichrysum is such an expensive oil. Over recent years there have been several failed harvests which made it very difficult to meet growing demand of new markets.

Chemistry

In a moment, we will look at the chemistry profiles of some of the most popular sources of Helichrysum italicum. Before we do though, I thought it might be useful to look at what you might be able to expect some of the principle components to do, then it will make it easier to look at a GC report knowing what you are looking for. As you go through the chemistry you will see that the essential oils vary from country to country but actually also region to region. The essential oils are, to all extents and purposes almost like completely different plants.

Corsican Helichrysum has high amounts of beta-diones (also known as di-ketones of italidones). These are rarely found in nature and are linked to spiritual and physical healing. They are useful for all kinds of depression, nervous exhaustion, lethargy and stress. You will see later that they also have the effects of moving energy and physical matter as in the case of refusing to let blood pool in haemotoma.

Curcumene is antiseptic and extremely good at taking on inflammation. It is reputed to be even more anti-inflammatory than *Camomile matricaria*.

Neryl acetate is a very good skin healer but we would also see it indicated for stiff joints, muscle contraction, and when you read the metaphysical you'll see what I mean by both types of pain in the neck!

Neryl acetate is, of course an ester and esters work very well with problems which involve acetylcholine. As the ester binds to the acetylcholine receptor site it inhibits its action, slowing it. Hence why you would see a relaxation as the muscle contraction slows. Apart from softening the muscles, acetylcholine is involved in inflammation, in particular redness of the skin and blushing, fatigue from exertion, gall bladder problems.

Low levels of acetylcholine contribute to consistently high levels of inflammation cause pain, atherosclerosis, hypercoagulation (easy blood clotting) and premature aging. You can also expect to see fast pulse and dilated pupils.

In short it affects every system in the body that has something to do *unconsciously*. So heartrate, breathing digestion etc. etc.

As you might expect from these, it is also affected by the emotions. People with low acetylcholine levels will often suffer with the inability to cope with their emotions. Their emotional state can be unpredictable.

An oil that is high in esters it is very gentle and tremendously calming and healing

There is a very interesting paper: *Chemical composition, antimicrobial activities and odor descriptions of some essential oils with characteristic floral-rosy scent and of their principal aroma compounds* by The University of Vienna which analyses how essential oils with a floral profile perform medicinally. *Jirovetz et al described the fragrance as being:* Fresh-piney, floral (rose- and orange-blossom-like), fruity (lemon notes), weak herbal-woody side-notes.

Their sample showed a chemistry of: Neryl acetate (12.2%), nerol (9.6%) and neryl propionate (4.8%) – further main components: α-Curcumene (20.7%), α- pinene (17.8%), β-caryophyllene (5.9%), γ-elemene (5.1%), limonene (3.2%), β-selinene (3.1%) and italicene (3.1%);

They were able to demonstrate that essential oils with floral-rosy scent, such as Helichrysum, but also citronella, geranium, palmarosa, rose and Verbena have high antimicrobial action against various microorganisms "*these effects are mainly the result of a combination of some also biologically active principal aroma compounds (geraniol, nerol, citronellol and many of their derivatives) in a medium up to high concentration."*

So we know that if we see any of these compounds in high quantities, we are likely to see very strong anti-microbial behaviours.

Chemotypes of Helichrysum italicum essential oil

This could be a book in itself because the changes are so diverse it is incredible. The way that the plant adapts and alters to its changing environment, soil and weather is like nothing you have ever seen.

I am just going to pick out a few research papers because there are literally hundreds on this aspect of the plant (so they can work out where best to extract their molecules from, I would suggest).

So let's have a look from the highest point of the cliff tops and see what we can see.

Corsican Helichrysum

First we can see Corsican producers who have to get a license to distil and export each year because helichrysm is so closely regulated by the government on Macquise.

They produce two types of oil: cultivated and wild harvested. The majority of oil produced is cultivated for the cosmetic industry. Wild harvested is on the decline but if you can get it the best oil comes from dry mountains in the south.

The typical profile looks like this:

a large presence of oxygenated compounds such as neryl acetate, neryl propanoate, nerol , acyclic ketones and β diketones.

If you are looking to buy a Corsican Helichrysum ideally you want your GC report to say you have least 30% neryl acetate, and italidione ranging from 8–12%.

Tuscan Helichysum

The Tuscan is higher in hydrocarbons such as α-pinene, β-caryophyllene, α & β selinenes

Let's compare the Corsican profile to what the University of Pisa had found from their samples of essential oils from Elba (Tuscany Italy). These were taken at three times throughout the year, in January, May October.

In total 115 constituents were identified which constitute 96.8-99.8% of the oil (so there is a tiny number of chemicals still to be identified and classified).

The main one found in the Elba samples was nerol. That constituted anything from 2.8-12.8* depending on location and the time of year the sample was taken. (Just it is not obvious, producers aim to harvest when the oil content is at its highest, which is July and then about September / October time). Next was its famous ester derivative neryl acetate that made up between 5.6-45.9% of the oil.

Croatian Helichrysum

Croatian is more similar to Italian origin. When it was analysed in an experiment in 2006, they were able to identify a minimum of 27 esters, but they suspected there were possibly more in various developmental stages because of the way that acids and alcohols form to create esters and the fact that when they had analysed before the fractional distillation only six had presented themselves.

However, as you will see life is never as simple as it seems...because there is enormous diversity between the oil profiles even from Croatia, depending on where it has grown.

In 2015, Palacky University in the Czech republic analysed the chemical constitents of Croation Helichrysums.

They took samples from BraČ Island, famed from its horseshoe shaped white pebble beach and found that the primary active component was α-trans-bergamotene (10.2%) and β-acoradiene (10.1%),. Leave the little island and travel just three hours to Biokovo Mountain and the profile looked very different. It was rich with neryl acetate, measuring as much as 8.1% of the total profile. β-acoradiene was a principle component in a sample taken in Tijaica, but in Makarsha rosifoliol was the richest making up 8.5% of the oil. Without getting into the specifics of exactly what each constituent might be expected to do, even to the uninitiated it is easy to see that the medicine of the plant from the mountain is not going to be the same as the one which grew near the glorious white beach.

Sardinian Helichrysum

Corsican and Sardinian are almost similar with dominating profiles of neryl acetate, nerol, neryl propinoate and linalool.

It makes me smile to think of the poor ethnobotanists sent out in the 1990s, to far flung places, trying to learn how the healers of the area used their plants. I should think anyone that brought home details about Helichrysum would have got the sack. They would have had a list of uses and very little understanding of just how important it would be to choose the exact bush, under the specific tree, next to a particular river, near to where Cleo the chameleon danced last week! Poor guys, they did not stand a chance!

Moral of the story...have a look at a GC report before you buy. It should always be available upon request.

Ethnobotany

It would seem to me that Helichrysum has been an essential ingredient for herbalists across the world and whilst there is very little historical data to draw on from Europe, strangely historical evidence from Africa has plenty to say. As we would expect there is a great deal of difficulty in identifying exactly which species of Helichrysum is being used, but much work has been done by ethnobotanist into allocating species and also parts used in each case.

Many different chemotypes of Helichrysum are used throughout Southern Africa in their traditional medicines. The documented medicinal use of Helichrysum can be traced back to 1727 by a Dutch Physician called Boerhaave.

Boerhaave was a celebrated physician and botanist. He is considered to be the founder of clinical medicine having been the first person to see the connection between symptoms and lesions. He is also the first person to be able to isolate urea from urine. It was he that noted that one particular Helichrysum species was used to treat nervousness and hysteria. Where his knowledge of that initially came from is not known. It may have been derived from knowledge gained from the local Khoi and San peoples, but there has also been some speculaton that European botanists used their knowledge of medicinal properties of their European genera and then translated them across (Scott and Hewett, 2008). I wonder, then, does this give us a better insight into 18th Century European usage? It is impossible to tell.

Common names:

kooigoed, sewejaartjie(Afrikaans); ***everlastings*** (Englis h); ***phefo-ea-loti***, ***toanae-moru*** (Southern Sotho); ***imphepho***(Zulu); ***phefu***, ***isicwe*** (Xhosa).

Sewejaartjie means last for seven (sewe) years (jaar) when kept in the house. Usually this more refers to the papery flowers that we find in dried flower wreaths. The prefix geel is sometimes added and it means yellow.

The leaves and stems of the European Helichrysum gymnocomum & H. herbaceum are burned as incense to ensure the goodwill of the ancestors.

Helichrysum nudifolium is used by the South African ***Xhosa*** people to treat circumcision wounds and is known as *isicwe*. Again this is used as incense for the ancestors. This also forms part of the Zulu tradition.

Medicinally the cultures also use our *italicum* for chest complaints, colic, fever, coughs, colds and headaches. I was interested to find they also revere it for internal sores, which I probably would not have thought of it for but actually it makes perfect sense to me.

Medicinally, the roots, leaves, stem and flowers of the African Helichrysum are used for a variety of complaints and ailments. Depending on the species and where it grows, uses include: angina pectoris, backache, bladder conditions, coronary thrombosis, coughs, colds, circumcision wounds, eye complaints, fever, infected sores, heart conditions and weakness, high blood pressure, 'flu, kidney infections, painful periods, rheumatism, urinary infections, and to prevent infection. It is one of their foremost medicines for virility and wound-healing but is also beloved for its insect repellent abilities. These can be seen in Dioscoride's assertion that laying the herbs amongst your clothes prevents them from being eaten by moths or worms.

The following information is taken from the Royal Museum of Central Africa Plants Database

Helichrysum odoratissimum:

The juice of the leaves used as drops in eyes for conjunctivitis,

The leaves are used as a decoction for pregnant women when the "foetus don't move", and also for anaemia.

Leaves in a water infusion for a cough

Infusion of the leaves: psychosis and to rid of bad spirits .

The following is taken from "*Plants of Xhosa people in the Transkei region of Eastern Cape (South Africa) with major pharmacological and therapeutic properties*" by R. B. Bhat

Helichrysum appendiculatum Less. (RBB 78) *"Isicwe"*

Fresh leaves are used as an antiseptic to speed healing after surgery but also after circumcision cutting to prevent external inflammation. Crushed leaves are also used as a bandage on the sores and wounds caused by hot water or fire

Helichrysum cymosum D.Don (RBB 249) "Impepho"

The leaves are boiled in water and the decoction is used to cure headache. It is also used to drive away the evil spirits from home

Helichrysum leiopodium DC. (RBB 269) letapiso

Entire plant is used. The fresh leaves are boiled in water and the hot lotion is used to bathe swollen feet for rapid recovery

Helichrysum nudifolium Less. (RBB 93)IColocolo

A handful of leaves are boiled in water and the fumes are inhaled directly for the treatment of cold and flu.

Ubiquitous at all gatherings of izangoma to summon the ancestors. To cleanse relationships and to draw on the authority of the ancestors.

Helichrysum stenopterum

It is used by women to wash away body odours while *Helichrysum cooperi Harv.* is used as a wash by young men wishing to attract women (Watt & Breyer- Brandwijk 1962). *Helichrysum odoratissimum* (L.) Sweet is used by the Sotho to fumigate huts and to make a pleasantly perfumed ointment (Watt & Breyer-Brandwijk 1962).

The Sotho tribe living in the south use it to fumigate their huts. They mix it with fats to make a sweet ointment which was reputedly only allowed to be worn be the wives of the Chiefs. They rub the ashes of the burn leaves into wounds to prevent scarring. Vomiting is eased by eating these ashes.

It is burned as an incense to conjure the protection and benevolence of the incestors. The smoke is also reputed to chase away demons and possession as well as "curing" insanity. The Xhosa also use the plant in their spiritual practices, using it as a cleansing and strengthening fumigant when a baby is born.

The smoke is inhaled as a sedative, and is believed to protect whomsoever it touches. Inhaling the smoke of the leaves is reputed to ease headaches.

They make a sweet tea from the flowers and leaves to ease tension, cramps and nervous energy and to invite sleep. This is also used treat colic and also the stitch! They use a decoction to treat abdominal pain, and also one of the leaves to ease febrile convulsions.

Female sterility is treated by drinking a decoction of the leaves and twigs, and once pregnant these women continue to drink their elixir as a tonic to help them through their pregnancy. Once healthily delivered this decoction helps to bring in and strengthen their milk flow.

The root is boiled and used to treat colds and coughs. These are also treated by eating the ash made from the twigs. It is used as a "cathartic purgative" – whether this is only to remedy the bowels or to induce some kind of profound emotional release, I cannot tell.

Juice squeezed from the leaves and stems is used as eye drops for conjunctivitis. This is also used to treat heartburn and flatulence.

Extract of the flowers is used to treat dehydration (although I can't quite identify how that is prepared).

In Rwanda, Helichrysum is used to treat both menstrual pain and eczema.

Lastly the stems and flowers are used a soft bedding material for the cattle offering the extra bonus of being an effective insect repellent.

This information is sourced from: South African Helichrysum species: A review of the traditional uses, biological activity and phytochemistry: A.C.U. Lourens et al.

The Metaphysical Aspects of Helichrysum's Healing

Archetype

Every book presents me with its own set of challenges and this section is Helichrysum's. As previously stated there is very little knowledge to draw on, because of strange changes of name but also the apparent non-usage before the 1980s.

In some authorities it is cited as being under Sun rulership and with such strengthening medicine, that would seem to be absolutely true, and yet...something feels like it is missing.

Others cited Jupiter and given its benefits on diabetes and cholesterol, I felt happy with this. But yet a doubt kept niggling. Mars often arises often in the Victorian Herbals, and since Artemis has such strong associations with battle, that too seemed to be a jigsaw piece that was in the right puzzle but in the wrong place. For weeks, this festered in my mind. It seemed to me that Saturn must be in play, because it had such strong associations with skin, but again, the medicine would not fit. Then I had a thought. What if it could not have been satisfactorily classified by the Ancients because they had not discovered its planet? What about Pluto or even Neptune?

But no.

And then I recalled a story of a healer that had been trained by Artemis...A centaur no less, and the entire story of the healing seems to fit perfectly.

I propose that *Helichrysum italicum* be classified similar to how clary sage is ruled by mercury and the moon, by two planets jointly. For clary sage, the internal communication systems (Mercury) are affected by the emotions (moon) in the menstrual cycle and during menopause. Even the impact of Alzheimer's from a women's history with hot flushes then can be influenced by the relationship between Mercury and the Moon.

I lay before you that our new friend Helichrysum may perhaps fall under Chiron's rulership because of its relationship to the Sun. Pray, grant me several minutes of your time to explain my reasoning.

Firstly, recall Kurt Schnaubelt's very astute testimony about Helichrysum...something I had not even noticed before. That there are no mentions of Helichrysum in any aromatherapy text books before 1980.

1st November 1977 10am, Charles T Kowal reviewed photographs taken on October 18th. Astrological writer Eric Francis explains that "though Chiron was finally discovered in 1977, pre-discovery photos exist from as early as 1895. In other words, though it had been photographed repeatedly by observatories, it was not actually noticed, catalogued and named untill nearly a century later."

Kowal had pinpointed a previously *unobserved* minor planet that orbits between Saturn and Uranus. Although it is classified as a minor planet, it is also believed to be both a comet and an asteroid. Chiron was the first member of a new class of cosmic objects to be identified which are now known as centaurs. These bodies orbit between the asteroid belt and the Kuiper belt, (a stellar disc of the Solar System,) way beyond the planets, extending from Neptune's orbit to the Sun.

These massive distances are calculated in AU, denoting *Astronomical Units*. One Astronomical Unit represents approximately the distance of the Earth to the Sun. Chiron is calculated to be 30AU around Neptune to approximately 50 AU from the Sun. Chiron and another centaur (with the slightly less memorable name: 10199 Chariklo), are the only other bodies in the Solar System (apart from the four major planets, Saturn, Uranus, Jupiter and Neptune) known to have rings.

In Greek mythology Chiron was centaur and was the son of Saturn. He was born of an elicit encounter between the cheating god and Philyra, a sea nymph in Thessally. Saturn's wife Rhea came across them during their interlude and Saturn being the fine upstanding guy he was, decided to hide from her and changed himself into a stallion right at the moment of climax. (*I dunno about you, but that would really put me off my stride?)* Anyway the result of this bizarre union was a being who was half mortal, half immortal and strangely half man, half horse (but also some portion of sea creature, I suppose, if you can forgive the maths).

Legend has it, he was the first born of the centaurs, but even in this light he was different. Other centaurs had the upper body of a man and the lower body of a horse having been born of Sun and cloud (Ixion and Nephele) but Chiron's front legs were also human signifying his superiority over his species. In short, he was a species, all alone.

Immediately, on setting eyes upon the bestial baby she had produced, his mother walked away from him and turned herself into a tree, abandoning Chiron, in the hope he might die at the top of Mount Pelion. He would have, of course, had he been mortal but the immortal part of his being prevented this from happening. The equine nature of the beast naturally thrived on the mountain's rocky slopes. Chiron began his life isolated, alone and marginalised nevertheless, he was successful in raising himself.

Chiron was a sensitive, gentle and patient creature, completely dissimilar to the rest of his kind. The centaurs were hell raisers, drunks and sodomisers; we often see them depicted in Ancient Greek pottery and literature representing barbarism and unbridled chaos. It should be stated here though, that the centaurs, as a race get a pretty bad press, because they are often shown in this light in the myths but in each case it is when they are under the influence of wine. It seems to always be the booze that is always their undoing.

In time, Artemis and her twin brother Apollo discovered the lonely centaur on the hillside. They adopted him as their own and housed him in a cave on Mount Pelion. There, he was able to live in peace and to study many things as well as marry his consort and have many children. Under the tutelage of Apollo, he learned ethics, philosophy, mathematics, music, reason, logic and medicine; in short all that is redeeming about civilization. Artemis taught him the ways of the forest, the use of herbs and all that is important about the wilderness and nature. She taught him to hunt with spectacular archery skills as well as her guardianship of young children. Chiron was a great student absorbing every lesson he was ever given. *This* was the skill that would eventually lead to his glory.

By and by, Chiron became famed for his ability to pass on his knowledge and skills which he shared generously. These gifts stood him in great stead in his vocation of training young boys to become outstanding men, which he was often called upon to do.

For instance, an occasion arose when Apollo impregnated Cronus but found that she had been subsequently been unfaithful to him. Incandescent with rage he sent his sister Artemis to avenge him, ordering her to kill Cronus, which she did. Apollo felt a little guilty and cut open her belly and rescued his unborn child from within. (This is thought to have been the world's first caesarean delivery). The child, Asclepius, was given to Chiron to train in his cave. Here, Chiron taught him all the secrets of healing using plants and herbs. Over time Asclepius became a *far superior* doctor and is considered the father of medicine. Ancient engravings also show pictures of Asclepian manipulation which also leads to the theory that Chiron may also have taught him the bone manipulation techniques that carry his name *chiropractice*. Other students included famous heroes of the Greek myths, such as Achilles, Theseus, Jason, Peleus, Perseus, and Hercules.

Chiron trained the heroes with the skills required for their adventures. To Jason, he gave the skills of navigating the stars, for him to find the Golden Fleece and he had prepared Hercules for his 12 labours with many gifts including how to make a lethal poison arrow. One day Hercules was visiting another of the centaurs. Pholus (also thought to have been civilised) had offered him food and a few days' rest from his labours. They had supper and Hercules asked for wine. This was quite a shocker for Pholus, who ate his meat raw, but he considered the request. Dionysus had given him vessel of sacred wine some time ago, to be kept in trust by the centaurs until the right time arose for its opening. To ingratiate

Hercules's wishes, Pholus was forced to produce the vessel. The hero, desperate for wine to wash down the raw meat, grabbed it from him and forced it open. The fragrance was beguiling and delicious. It drifted out of the cave and danced on the nose of every centaur surrounding them. Each was lured to the cave and joined the party but as the drinking continued the centaurs became more and more lairy. Soon, they were attacking Hercules in a bid to seize the sacred wine for themselves. Hercules reacted using his poisoned arrows. Quietly watching the furore was Chiron, who on seeing all of the slaughtered centaurs around him was fascinated to see what had caused their demise. He picked up one of the arrows, inspected it and then accidentally dropped it onto his foot, presumably then realising what it contained.

Ovid tells us in Fastis:

> *While the old man fingers the foul, poisoned shafts,*
>
> *An arrow slips out and stabs his left foot.*
>
> *Chiron groaned and hauled the iron from his flesh* (5.397-99)

The pain was excruciating and relentless but of course, that which should have been a gift, his immortality, immediately became his curse. All around him, lay dead centaurs, but for him here was no end to the searing pain. For nine days Chiron desperately laboured over his herbs and potions trying to find a poultice or salve that would ease the agony, but despite his healing knowledge, the wound would not heal.

Day and night he had to bear it, until finally he could. He hatched a plan to strike a bargain to end his pain.

He knew of the great torture befalling a Titan by the name of Prometheus. A clever trickster, Prometheus had stolen fire from the gods, given it as a gift to man, and then taught him how to use the gift showing them metalwork. Zeus was furious and set about punishing the Titan by chaining him to a rock and sending a vulture, daily, to chew out his liver. Titans were immortal so he could not die and the next morning, his liver had always grown back (Is it only me that thinks the fact that liver regrowth in a three thousand years old myth is rather chilling and insightful?!) and so the fear and torture never ended.

Hercules eventually came upon Prometheus in his eleventh labour and shot down the vulture with his poisoned arrows. His torture was over, but the creator of mankind remained shackled to his pillar or rock. Hercules could not bear to see how he had not ended the pain, merely changed it, and so begged Chiron to help him find a way to free him. Chiron saw an opportunity and begged Zeus for mercy, to allow Prometheus to be freed, and in payment he would offer up his own immortality. The bargain was struck that as long as he was needed as a trainer of demigods, he would exist in this world. Zeus agreed.

Finally, with a weeping Achilles looking on, Zeus honours his promise. Prometheus is freed and Chiron passes into the stars. He remains in the constellation of Sagittarius for our remembrance and inspiration whenever we need it.

Medical Astrology of Chiron.

Chiron governs **Wounds That Will Not Heal. M**ore than that, it represents that quintessential decision as to whether we live or die. It's a strange reality that a person can undergo such extensive injuries that they *should* die, and yet something inside them refuses to let it be so. They defy science and explanation. Theirs are the tales of miracles. In the same way, men together on the battlefield fight side by side and sustain the same grotesque injuries. The first can recover in mind but the other is lost to the oblivion of PTSD. This is Chironic medicine, the ability to hold on, to bear the weight of wounds which will not heal.

There is a sad irony in the centaur's tale but in many cases it is misconstrued by optimistic interpreters, and in doing so they miss a vital point of the learning. They relate it was through his pain that he became a healer, but that is a shallow misinterpretation. He did not become a healer *through* his pain, he *already was one*. The paradox was that, in the end that served him poorly. He could not fall back onto his innate abilities because this time, they were simply not enough.

Psychologically we can say that Chiron represents our deepest wound **and our efforts to heal that wound**. It speaks of our experience of pain, alienation and woundedness but also the rainbow bridge we finally crossed to find our way out of it. Often that wound might be a psychological one or in the Centaur's case, of course, a more physical one. This is most certainly the medicine of Helichrysum. Not only will it help to heal the skin to a level beyond compare to other plants, but it is able to talk to the darkest part of the soul that very dearly wants to give up.

There might be a Pollyanna temptation to imagine that it can create magic and force our beloveds to remain with us on this mortal plane, but I do not think that is so. Rather it sings its sanctuary song, whispering:

"I will be with you until you have had enough. When that time comes, I'll help you to not be afraid. 'Till then, let's not worry about the things that have passed. Let me help you to carry the weight of your burden. Let's take this one step at a time."

What burden?

Well, that is a complex issue and one that I have debated long and hard whether to include at depth or not. However, I suspect this might be the very first essential oil to be categorised under Chiron's rulership (although if I am right then there must be many more to be found). In that case then, it makes sense to include it. My apologies to those who don't like the metaphysical, I shall try to keep the portions of the book as separate as I can so you can skip it if you want to.

For those of you who are interested, I'd like to direct you to the beautiful work of Liz Greene about Chiron and his place in medical astrology. It was her work that inspired me to think that this maybe a good rulership.

Liz Greene sees Chiron as essential in deepening our understanding of solar consciousness; for in order to choose to live life to the full, we have to face that part in us that would rather seek death.

This will to live is an enigma. We may passionately cry our proclamation that we want to live; but somewhere deep inside, the soul longs to go home. No matter how quietly it whispers, this yearning for oblivion has the capability to overpower any conscious desire for treatment to work. Why is it, we must wonder, that a set of people might react to conflict, to pain and to disappointment with some kind of new perspective that metamorphoses their outlook where others are swallowed by bitterness. Hopeless, they are unable to see the colours of joy we perceive and instead inhabit some kind of grey twilight world. Worse, over time, each day merges into a new version of Hell, so they beg for it to end and eventually find their will to live misplaced.

There is a strange synchronicity to these deaths, I think too. Not only do we include deliberate suicides with very clear cut intention here, but also those “accidents” of the heartbroken that make you wonder, what if? Unconscious actions, most definitely. But was the subconscious seeking to pull a blanket over this existence after screaming in silence for so long? With Chirons transits we might find self-destructive behaviour, addictions, self sabotaging and probably downright self hatred. So just as we wonder at where that spark of self will might hide inside of us, we might also ponder why some “survivors” still endeavour to destroy themselves whilst others are content to lash out and scar those people around them. I am sure many of us can identify with a person hurting so deeply they make everyone around them a scapegoat for their pain.

With any polarity in life, we, as medical astrologers, always need to look at a polarity of planet. That is how the planets seem to speak to each other as their energies communicate through the solar system. Here we are searching for a relationship that influencing polarity of hope versus despair. Perhaps even the will to live versus hopelessness. To me, the relationship that creates this the strongest, is between the Sun and Chiron.

There is a danger in identifying any plant under one rulership, in the same way there is a danger to using standard essential oils recipes for every single patient...in that it does not bring the entire mind body spirit perspective into play. In fact, I have never seen this as clearly as whilst I have written this book. The interplay between Chiron and other planets makes it far easier to understand the medicine that we yield.

So, there are two very important relationships we must embrace here, the first is the relationship between Saturn and Uranus and the second is between Chiron and the Sun.

The entirety of medical astrology depends on the Sun being the ego of the person – that is his conscious active personality and **how that relates to the trials and challenges** that other planets present him with. (You might remember how Jupiter was to do with lessons of authority (Holy Basil), and Saturn with restriction (Spikenard), and Pluto being transformation (Vetiver)?)

Medical Astrology of The Sun

There is a great deal written about Sun medicine so I am not going to labour the point. Very quickly:

It rules the vital force of the body. Its main principle is the heart and circulation. In Chinese Medicine the Sun is seen to rule Shen which is the timeless aspect of a person, and in so doing it helps them to connect to their place in the collective consciousness. It is the sense of "I"-ness. It is the ego.

Sun medicine is strengthening and provides fortitude and resilience. It provides warmth and has a drying aspect. It assists anything that has a connection to circulation.

It brings about vigour and robustness. In addition, the Sun rules the back.

Helichrysum's Healing Journey Through Chiron

We think of how Chiron transits through space. It exists between Saturn and Uranus and because of its strange ellipse, might sometimes even travel as far out as near to Neptune.

Try to think of the travelling it does, almost as weather systems it must face. On much of its journey, it cannot absorb the creative energy of the Sun because it is too far away. Saturn is sending gusts of restriction and fear. Somehow he has to find a way to get to the transformative energy of Pluto whilst navigating the shocks and upsets that Uranus likes to send its way.

In our astrological life, it is only by travelling with Chiron through his lessons from Saturn's restriction that we can reach Pluto's transformation.

So how?

Well, Chiron's medicine is unusual because his innate ability is not what it seems to be. It is not his healing that is his salvation. It is his consistent learning and sharing, his imparting of knowledge, that is. It is not Chiron that is considered the God of Medicine, it is his student Aesclepius. The lesson is that perhaps we may be "disabled" (dreadful word choice, sorry) but we still have enormous amount to teach. We must find purpose in our suffering and use it to create something good. Perhaps there *is* no way out of the pain we have, but we have other gifts to give and many things to learn from our days living in that pain.

There is no physical representation of Chiron medicine, as such. Not in the same way that Venus is the heart or Jupiter the liver, anyway. What we have instead is this over-arching theme of *Wounds That Will Not Heal* which encompasses everything, in a way doesn't it? That could be tissue, bones, organs or even emotional damage. In the next section, I'll lay out which houses in the chart rule each part of the body and that makes it easier to understand, but for now think "It could be anything that will not heal..."

Chiron transits between the outer planets, so his messages and his challenges are nothing to do with the actual identity of the *individual* (because that comes from the planets closer to the Sun), the ones you see with Chiron <u>are ancestral or ones that were brought with the individual into their incarnation</u>. This need not actually be from past life, we might say familial, societal, cultural or even ethnicity for example, these issues belong to the collective. Whatever the context, the important thing to note is these are things that *cannot* be changed. By their nature these are not necessarily wounds that *will* not heal, more that they are *un*healable. Again when we get to the houses, you will understand this more.

As with any other horoscope factor, Chiron has a positive as well as a negative side. For one thing, it shows where we may teach and help others. It shows where we can do things better for others than we can for ourselves. Chiron shows where we can have an affinity for teaching, but, ironically, that is where we can teach others how to do things *better than we can* do them ourselves.

At this point it might be interesting for you to know that I have Chiron in just about the most prominent place in my chart. I have him in the first house and also 3 degrees after my ascendant so it is also my rising planet. I am a healer, but what I have found I am good at is teaching other people ways to use their healing. (Incidentally, most of the rest of my planets are in the 8th house which rules publishing!)

Now, remember I said that you will hear it told that it is *through* his suffering he becomes a great teacher. But that is *not true* is it? *(Can you hear me growling?!)* Because Chiron already was an incomparable teacher, *so* revered was he, that the gods brought their loved ones to him. More, one could say that he was already wounded *even before* the arrow struck him. The poor centaur was born different from his kind, was abandoned by his mother, was ostracised and had to raise himself alone. He is neither man nor beast and yet he's both. He belongs in no world. The lesson in the archetype might indeed be that there is lesson in the pain...and that would entirely be true and the lesson must be learned but actually it is more that.... simply life is not fair.

In 21st century lingo...

Shit Happens. Deal with it.

And it's a vile lesson, especially to people like you and I who want to believe that the world is a good place and that good things happen to good people but the truth is that life's a bitch. The end.

But actually it's only the beginning, isn't it, because **Chiron is the process of the soul's awakening.**

It's a strange lesson, because on the surface it looks like a bad one and make no mistake, these are hard lessons, but Chiron lessons are also opportunistic and Helichrysum really helps to shine the Sunlight on that. Often the lesson will be bolt out of the blue, it will be sudden and explosive. That's the impact of Uranus at play.

Completely unexpected. Totally unreasonable and frankly, quite often it is an absolute f**ker. But it forces to you stop and take stock. And when we do, well, this is when the good stuff happens.

Jessica Garfield-Kabbar describes how Chiron's lesson is a paradox. The healer could not heal himself and also that poison of the medicine we have to swallow may also come to be our gift. She portrays how it is **our *relationship* with the substance that dictates whether it is a healer or a poison**, not the substance or circumstance itself.

The Shamanic Medicine man is often born from these Chironic trials, in particular near death experiences. You might see parallels with the therapists who decide to counsel because they are near to explosion with personal insights into pain and crazy! Their only way to ease the pressure they feel they are under is to help other people with theirs. It's like they have this to keep the pain close to them. Rather than trying to cure it, they take care of it, nurture and tend it. Perhaps they worry if they lose sight of it then they also lose control of it maybe? Who knows. What is clear, though, is they emanate grace from their wound truly helping others who feel the same to come to terms with their pain. Healing and helping has become their coping mechanism.

That's a long way down the road though isn't it? How does the veteran who comes back from war, shell shocked and damaged, get to be the person that holds another in empathy, teaching him the way back to the light? Therein lies the question doesn't, it? Certainly *this* is the rainbow bridge that we spoke about. The hardest part of Chironian medicine is to face the parts of ourselves that repulse us the most. We are required to reveal those parts we may have masked *all of our lives* for fear that, if only people knew, they would never want to be anywhere near us. There is a heavy requirement to face these feelings of inadequacy, to understand and embrace them and to forgive ourselves them.

Easy on paper.

These feelings of inadequacy and low self-worth, though, are fertile breeding grounds for addiction and self destructive behaviours. We start to recognise repeating patterns and repetitive compulsions, where the seems to be need to undo ourselves and despite the outcome never being very good, we have to go back to the bottle/bed/needle more and more often. Not only that but we need more and more. More whisky, more crack, another role of a dice to win back everything we have lost. Anything to block the pain, in the hope that life might just look a little better in the morning. But, of course, life does not work that way. All we end up is dirtier in the gutter, ashamed with a stinking, splitting head.

Worse, each time our spectacular displays of behaviour escalates, the chasm of the wound seems to be split deeper and wider. The threads of our behaviour affect and intersect with ever more people and pretty soon we have woven this smothering fabric of pain and destruction. This is the shadowside of Chiron. These are the clues that will lead us to a prescription of a person needing Helichrysum. What we need is to find a way to radiate the Sun onto the pained face to transmute the energy. Helichrysum's solar medicine does this. He opens the curtains and lets the light shine in.

This relationship with the Sun is absolutely essential to understanding the healing of Helichrysum. (And let's be fair here, a yellow plant named after the Greek Sun god Helios has to be a Sun medicine...)

The Sun is our certain special essence. It's the way we were incarnated on this particular plane at this time. More importantly it is the *purpose* of our inhabiting this plane. It is what we were born to be. It's through the Sun, that we perceive ourselves to be completely special and unique. It's the Sun's medicine that gives us a sense that we are part of something bigger, a part of something eternal. It is our sense of connectedness.

But, of course, consciousness is a bitch. It is painful and shocking and often that sense of disconnect can be fearful and traumatic. (The more traumatic the event that has disconnected us, the easier it is to blame God or even refuse to believe that he can exist at all.) Our soul's journey is always to be striving towards that sense of coming back to the Sun. Just like physical Sunshine, it gives us hope, a spring in our step and a sense that we are achieving something in life. When the Sun is aspected, then all's right with the world.

The clear themes of the Sun are: one's individual destiny, a clear sense of meaning in life and hope for the future. There is self-confidence and generosity of spirit. A person has a clear sense of identity, set apart from his or her family or tribe. These Sun kissed creatures have this incredible power to create, and that comes from the Sun's gift of trust in that part of themselves to be able to do that, and to succeed. In the same way, they are playful. To me, the Sun is encapsulated not only by a strengthening medicine but, overall, by hope.

Let's compare that with what Chiron's impact can do to a person.

In a complicated and unhealable way, he raises failings and flaws to do with one's family or bigger collective. The problems with the history of the patient that *cannot* be changed in any way. The situation looks hopeless and impossible. Fighting seems useless. They are disillusioned. Every one of their ideals has faded and failed. The wounding or injury they have been exposed to is utterly inescapable. Its pain is relentless and scars every single aspect of their being. The damage is both physical and psychological in a permanently reciprocal loop. Bitterness and cynicism seeps from every pore and there is an abandonment of any desire to create or bring about change.

In short, they are depressed.

The reverse of the Chironic coin brings about compassion. Sympathy is transmuted into deep empathy for other people's pain. It's a wisdom that can *only* come from deeply visceral *personal* perspective on pain. Nurturing and caring for the pained helps our Chironic hero to gain insights and a closer more personal understanding of his own pain and this is very helpful.

If there is no help for Chiron from the Sun then depression looms. Confidence steals away and the patient starts to have an overwhelming sense of the permanency of damage he has sustained. They become cynical, but more, they have this ongoing expectation that any efforts they, or those around them have, will fail. Because they are defensive (and because as they quite rightly perceive life *has* dealt them a shitty blow,) they apportion blame and spite to everyone around them. Furthermore, in a bid to avoid some of the inadequacy they feel, they over compensate and inflate their own ego by belittling everyone around them. Faced with this vile outlook of their hopeless future, surrounded by people whom they have come to despise, it seems less and less useful to stay on this mortal plane and gradually, ever so slowly the will to live slips away.

But when we can find Sun medicines, that exalt Chiron, then that viewpoint changes. *The situation or the poison does not change, purely the way that the person views it.* These people find an untapped resource of patience within, but more importantly they develop this useful pearl-like wisdom from the grit of living their reality every single day. The Sun allows the lips to raise in a knowing smile as they see their own patterns of behaviour reflected back at them; they recognise their reactions which turned so poisonous as life peppered them with ever more spiteful blows. In the days when the sadness and melancholy descends a different perspective takes form. Not depression, nor self-pity but simply a deeper pattern of thought and feeling. Sometimes there may be insights but for the main, simply a mantra of

It is what it is.

And as I write this I am able to see this panning out day to day. I am currently very close to the wound of friend critically injured in a car accident. She is a lovely person bright, intelligent and feisty. The accident was dreadful and she sustained injuries beyond belief. Somehow she has pulled though. After suffering dreadful memory problems, she seems to be, for the most part, intact.

Further down the Chironic journey, we see TV screens full of the stupendous feats of the Rio Paralympians. Theirs is the same journey as the able bodied Olympians, years of training hard and successes and defeats, and yet one has to wonder what made the Sun shine on each of their Chironic medicines? What is it that makes their will to live so fierce that it defies science and the expectations of doctors? What stopped these superheroes from turning over and sobbing into their pillow and had them chasing the ecstasy of winning Olympic medals? How did they find a way to accept the human limits that were now their new realities but, really allow the awakening of their specialness to seep through every core of their being?

There is a beautiful book by Jan Kusmirek. I am not sure how many of you have read it. It's about carrier oils and its title has resonated with me through this section. It is called "Liquid Sunshine" and that feels entirely true of Helichrysum. I feel its rulership must undoubtedly be Chiron, but in terms of that activation of the will to live then it is the searing heat of the Sun in the crucible that transfigures the spirit.

So we need to identify what this certain *je ne sais quoi* must be, and I suppose it must be hope. Astrologically the sign for hope is the Sun.

As I stated previously, most people call Chiron the Wounded Healer, but others call his transit the Rainbow Bridge because of his bridging aspect between Saturn and Uranus. (Incidentally, remember Saturn was Chiron's father, but also Prometheus is Uranus in the Roman Pantheon and it was his liver that was pecked out.) If you think about the length of cycles here, Chiron has a very long transit and he is known as the Machiavellian Planet because he zips in and out of the other planets and so sometimes a transit may be years other times only months. His behaviour is very unpredictable and feels very similar to the self-sabotaging patterns we see with people suffering his medicine.

In total, Chiron takes about half a century (50.36 years) to orbit the Sun and so his return comes when you are between 50-51, but *Uranus* transits happen when you are between about 38-46 and the lessons that arise during this period of life are very useful for preparing for the onslaught of the wounded healer's lessons.

I am going through my Uranus transit now and it is a time of great soul searching. It's the point in our life when we look inward and really examine how we feel about the way we are living our lives. Are we happy that we are living a life that is authentic and has purpose? There is often a want to feel much, much freer and so you might see rather inappropriate choices of cars and, of course, this vibration is ripe for affairs and elicit liaisons. For many it manifests as the time of mid-life crisis, but for about a third of us the transit will be lived out in a more constructive way. We knuckle down. We really examine what we are putting out into the world. If the work has been done, then by the time Chiron comes it is not so hard to deal with his medicine. (That's what I am hoping anyway, my Chiron's return is 6 years away and counting...)

It is very hard not to see Chiron's medicine as bad and without a doubt getting your leg blown off by a landmine or being smashed to bits in a RTC cannot be construed in any other way.

To do so would be glib.

(Please do not take this to be a prediction of what is going to happen to you. I am using sweeping generalisations to illustrate a point. Everyone's lesson's will be different.)

But there is something in the quietness and isolation, for many people, that allows a little voice inside to say “I flaming hated that job anyway” and start to chuckle at the irony that perhaps the hell they were living may be easier to walk away from after all.

I may have said this before because it is something I believe to the very core of me now. Regular readers will know I started to write because I had been ill with a blood clot in my lungs and I had to find something to make ends meet and it just happened that someone wanted a person who knew a bit about aromatherapy to write some notes for them. The rest as they say, is history. I make light of how hard up we were but in truth we sold our house the day it was due to be reposessed thanks to the mortgage company’s solicitor holding the foreclosure off. They were dark times and yet both my husband and I feel it was the greatest gift we have ever been given because it was so freeing to know that even when we lost everything, we were still here! We still had each other, Goddess only knows how we ended up living in a nicer place but we did and we had our health back. It was terrifying and yet it brought us peace. The scar is there though and I feel sick to the stomach when I see people struggling for cash. I rarely pass someone sleeping on the streets without fetching them a sandwich or something warm to eat because to the core of me I radiate gratitude that I have moved on to a better place. I understand their fear and confusion because, whilst I have never slept rough, I thank Goddess that it was only through her grace that I was spared it.

Likewise, I feel fury to the pit of my stomach when I hear someone deride the beaten wife who has not yet had the courage to leave. Their staying doesn't make sense and yet unless you have been that woman you can never understand every other road leads to hell, so paralysed in fear you remain. Unless you have stood in that woman's broken stilettos there is no possible way you can understand her pain.

You might sympathise, but you can never empathise. In the beautiful words of Jessica Garfield-Kabbar it's through the wisdom of experience that it becomes a living prayer. The poison becomes a gift.

When I meditated on Helichrysum I picked up a vibration that I recognised. It was an emotion that resonated painfully, that I knew and understood, but I also was aware was not part of *me*. It was familiar and yet not my own. I identified it as a very uneasy guilt. I sense something very similar with Jupiter ruled oils like Holy Basil quite often. It seemed to speak of being in a position of authority and the dreadful burden of sending off a generation of children to war. I kept thinking of what it must have been like, to be someone like Winston Churchill, and to have a whole country's expectations upon your shoulders. To live day to day with the paradox of having all those young lives on your conscience and to know that it was a necessary evil to achieve your completely moral objective. It reminded me of watching Benedict Cumberbatch portraying Alan Turin in the Initiation Game. There is a dreadful scene where they have cracked the Enigma Code which means they know which ship the Germans are going to attack. Indeed, we find the awful truth that one of their team has a brother on that very ship but they realise that they must not save it. To do so would signal to the enemy that their secrets have been uncovered and instead they create this dark mathematical formula to calculate which ships to save and those ones to allow to perish, as a means to give the allies *just* enough advantage to win the war.

My heart broke when I watched that film for many, many reasons, and it will leave a lasting imprint. It seemed like the dreadful blackness of Jupiter, the downside of playing your advantage. But now I see that it is not Jupiter; it is Chiron and the synchronicity makes me shake to my core.

For the guilt is not of the commander that I had envisioned, but that of the trainer. Of the centaur whose destiny it was to train these heroes in the skills they need to take on their own destinies and then to wait at home and to simply hope that it has been enough. Because, if you look closely at them, the quests of the heroes were no less than those of our soldiers today. Their encounters are those same that haunt our twenty first century nightmares. Jason had the responsibility of saving the entire Minoan civilisation on his shoulders when he set off to find the Golden Fleece. Which atrocities, I wonder, did Chiron fear the most for him, Gorgons with serpent heads, three headed dogs guarding the gates of hell or that he might end up skewered in some muddy trench. As he coached his protégés, I wonder how many nights did he remain awake, wondering if he had done enough; if there could have been a way he could have taken their place. How many times had he wished that there was a way that he could have taken their places and spared them their own destinies? How hard was it, I wonder, to know that this was his lot and, rather than rail against it, to accept it and find a way to bear it?

Perhaps it sounded something a little like this song written in E minor, the same key that Helichrysum vibrates on.

Five Finger Death Punch https://www.youtube.com/watch?v=o_l4Ab5FRwM

"*Right or wrong, I can hardly tell. I'm on the wrong side of heaven, the righteous side of hell*" On his darker days, in his cave, where the rays of the Sun god could not touch him, which side of the moral sword would Chiron consider he fell?

How close I wonder does it come to Gabriel Mojay's interpretation of the emotions courted by Helichrysum in his beautiful book *Healing the Spirit? "most indicated are enduring resentment, half-conscious anger, bitterness of spirit, and a stubbornly negative attitude."*

Four hooves, Chiron might have had, and animal instincts, but they came from below the waist. It was his *human* thinking self that sent those boys into battle. For those who consider us to be superior to animals, perhaps you might want to turn that around in your mind a little. I feel sure that perhaps he did.

Let's hear what conversations might take place in the lightless cover of the cave, as he considered what he had done sending Hercules out into his quest. He has first-hand experience of what could have happened if the Hydra had hurt his student on his second trial (the poison in his leg would be a conscious reminder), and so by the time Hercules reaches his 11th trial, meeting the vulture gnawing at Prometheus's liver Chiron must be descending into the bowels of madness and worry. Is it his fault? What can he do to stop it? How can he end this eternal stream of sacrifice of young lives?

10, 000 people, maybe more....

"Hello Darkness, my old friend...."

Sounds of Silence – Disturbed https://www.youtube.com/watch?v=u9Dg-g7t2l4

The only way to end the suffering it is to offer himself up in sacrifice. Whichever way you look at it, his decision is Christ like and noble.

For some people, you can see how a stubbornly negative attitude might prevail. Perhaps even, it might seem to us, to be entirely appropriate for their lot. Often we can look at these people and think "There, but for the grace of God go I." Life seems to have dealt them the cruellest blows and it is easy to see why they might be bitter. And yet in our twenty first century emancipation, psychoneuroendocrinology shows what a corporeal catastrophe that can be. The neurons send acerbic messages of discontent to the organs and they rot us from the inside. One can hardly fail to notice the timespan of just four years between the discovery of the opiate receptor which was to herald the new understanding of the mind body connection and then the subsequent noticing of the planet astrologers deem to be "Holistic".

Perhaps we were simply not ready.

Not ready for the planet, or maybe not ready for the plant.

There seem to be two main authorities about Chiron: Barbara Hand Clow and Melanie Reinhardt. The strange thing is that I had a copy of Reinhardt and mum had Hand Clow's even though neither of us professed to have deep interest in Chiron.

Both books have been with the family for years, it seems, and yet they have merely gathered dust on our shelves. That seemed odd to me, but of course very useful in this instance!

Hand Clow says: "The significant work going on with modern healers, astrologers and teachers, is the teaching that we change the planet and future if we change ourselves: It is called the Great Work by alchemists."

Certainly if we can change our perception to the poison it will most definitely influence the future we are able to manifest. There is a tendency for people to see medical astrology as a glorified version of cataclysmic soothsaying; as a rather morbid sense of seeing into our physical futures, but that is not so. For us there is no fatefulness that must come true because as soon as we change our behaviour or our attitude to something, in other words ourselves, then future and reality changes too. So could it mean, I wonder, if the common man can not only control destiny and become a hero of their own tale, but that they ultimately become responsible for their own physical destiny too, for his/ her own health?

Barbara Hand Clow seems to think so. She writes: "Magic has always relied heavily upon secret word formula which are written down and the actual sighting of Chiron may hint at the power of the priesthood maybe over with. That anyone can learn the sacred sounds and words to the revelation of the secrets."

I wonder.

Sounds like what's happening to plant medicine to me. Out of the hands of the wise woman in the woods, into the hands of the common man.

Actually, it sounds like holistic medicine to me. And what is Chiron? He is the healer, the wounded and the warrior, he is entirely holistic. He is, in fact complementary/ alternative medicine.

And therein is the very cataclysm of Helichrysum learning. To know that some wounds will not heal and if that must be so, to find a way to bear them.

Addiction

Valerie Ann Worwood wrote in 1999 of Helichrysum *"It helps the walking wounded and those that cannot reminisce for fear of the painful emotions that may be remembered. Helichrysum's spiritual and transpersonal purpose is to make self-exposure safe"*. In the Fragrant Pharmacy she built on this and described how Helichrysum had been used to treat drug addiction and that had been extremely successful used alone (rather than in a blend). Likewise, she expresses how it is extremely useful after trauma because it also helps with amnesia, so would be indicated if there were some degree of numbness, shock or disbelief. She lists it as one of the oils she would choose if she wanted to instil joy but also the one she would choose to speak to the inner child.

Essentialoilspedia.com have a very interesting page where they cite different oils for specific addictions such as food and work. They offer Helichrysum as being useful against alcohol and pornography. They give no reasoning as to why though.

Addiction most certainly makes sense to me. When I first picked up the oil I could see war. Perhaps it was the vibration of the war that has so recently scarred Croatia that I saw. I could smell the dirt, the blood, the stench of fear. The darkness was obliterated by the brightness of fire and explosions rang in my ears. Most certainly this is a medicine for the traumatised and the numbed.

The statistics for substance users in cases of PTSD are terrifying. According to one study (Pietrzak et all 2011), 46.4% of individuals with lifetime PTSD also met criteria for a substance use disorder (SUD). In another (Kulka et al 1990), 27.9% of women and 51.9% of men with lifetime PTSD also had SUD. Horrifyingly, women suffering PTSD were 2.48 times more likely to meet prerequisites for alcohol abuse or dependence and it was 4.46 times likelier that they would also meet them for drug abuse or dependence than it would be for women without PTSD. Men were 2.06 times (alcohol) and 2.97 times (drugs) more likely.

Twice as likely for men and a horrifying 450% more likely if you are a woman that you will turn to drink or drugs.

The need to escape the pain on the unresolved trauma and the feelings of powerlessness are so profound that only an altered state will suffice. What a dark place of despair.

I feel like we are back in Chiron's cave again, licking the wound that just will not give us respite. In particular nightmares and flashbacks of PTSD usually involve crises that have never properly resolved in the person's psyche. You might think of the soldier, taken prisoner in conflict and was unable to fight his captors. We might find that his flashbacks of the incident are his mind's unique mechanism of working through the unresolved anger and fear.

Likewise, perhaps we might think of the vulnerable child feeling utterly powerless after being sexually abused by an older relative. We can see how he might grow up living with overwhelming feelings of helplessness and the need to take revenge and how this might keep stealing into his thoughts.

The most common causes of PTSD being co-morbid with addiction is a history of sexual abuse. Combat is another common reason for PTSD, and this is especially true for men. Between 60 and 80 percent of Vietnam veterans who seek help for PTSD also require treatment for substance abuse.

Just as a footnote: Just as a in case any of you feel you would like to use Helichrysum for addiction problems. In Essential Aromatherapy: A Pocket Guide to Essential Oils and Aromatherapy by Susan Worwood and Valerie Ann Worwood, suggests that essential oil usage should be ***halved when treating the symptoms of addiction.***

Chiron in the natal chart

I promised that the medicine of Chiron in terms of what the person's burden might be, or indeed the physical manifestation of it could be, would become easier to understand when we got to learning what astrological house rules. So, here it is.

Welcome fellow metaphysical junkie. Come into the darkness of my cave. You have much to learn and I suspect when you have read this you will have a whole new thirst for knowledge because there is very little written about astrological aromatherapy and I find it fascinating and entirely useful. It is how mum began her quest in aromatherapy because she noticed that certain placements in people's charts would keep bringing up similar conditions so she set about finding ways to help all of the old people she had coming to see her, in pain, who could not get any relief from the doctors. That was how Jill Bruce Aromatherapy was born. It feels weird to have been steered right back onto her path. (Some might even say it was something to do with the history of the family, or my collective!)

Before I start, I want to acknowledge that I owe a great debt to four people for help with this section. They are Jean Wiley (if you want to talk about addictions, her Youtube channel is one of mine!), Melanie Reinhardt and Barbara Hand Clow. All of this work comes entirely from them and I am grateful to for their efforts and generosity. Lastly, but certainly not least to my mum Jill Bruce who has particularly navigated me through the minefield of the section you are about to read now.

Let's begin...

We talked a lot about transits in the medical astrology section so that pertains to moments in our life when Chiron passes a point in the sky that will communicate in some way with the other planets in our horoscope. But we also all have Chiron placed in our natal chart and this often profoundly affects our psychology as we traverse life. Whilst it has a placement in everyone's chart, it is not always placed *prominently* and, as such, means that it would not have such a damaging/ advantageous effect. It can be illuminating to see exactly where Chiron is placed in your own chart.

Since we are talking about helichrysum also being a Sun medicine here and Sun is always about the ego, I sense there will be a few of you with excited hands in the air going Me, Me, do me! Here's a link to plot yours before we begin.

http://www.astrologyonline.eu/Graphic/Form_Input/Input_Data_Chiron.asp

For transparency, Chiron is in my first house which is freakishly the healer and I suspect that, by the very nature of my readership, there will be a few more of you out there. (I predict at least 1 in 12!)

As we plot this position, it helps us to understand a lot about the karmic lesson that we came into this life with. It is like a collective burden of our ancestry that went before us. It might be carried from the experiences in the womb, from the psychology and situation of our parents or social group, or it might even be brought through from a past life, some would say. (*Or of course it could be religious/tribal and you might bear the mark of circumcision to prove it and then we already know Helichrysum helps that too...!)*

I think there might be a danger of viewing Chiron in an interminably dark light, but there is always a positive in these lessons, a kind of bonus gift if you like.

Chiron is the chart's healer. It travels around the chart like a doctor doing home visits. It offers healing opportunities to any planetary placement that presents itself. Sometimes, if the requirement for healing is really important, symptoms of the unhealthy planetary function will show themselves and flare up helping draw our awareness to its need for attention.

During Chiron transits, you will find mentors present themselves. Suddenly you find yourself surrounded by people whom you can emulate helping you to cultivate far healthier expressions of the parts of your personality you are seeking to heal.

So for example, when Chiron transits your Sun, self-esteem issues raise their heads. And because this is now an issue for you the Chiron transits often coincide with some kind of epiphany about the obstacles affecting you having confidence in yourself. Hopefully you then work on enhancing your own sense of worth and have the courage to accept the help of those around you. Then, of course we have the Chironic gift that when your self-concept is healthy and strong, Chiron might also present you that opportunity to pay that mentorship forward to others.

Because Chiron has such a strange ellipse, it is impossible to predict where it will be exactly in your chart without an ephemeris or some good astrology software. Even then you could only do it for each individual, whereas with Mars you can say he moves every two years or a Saturn return happens at 29 years. Except for Chiron’s return at 50-51 years, it is impossible.

In Aries, when it is at furthest from the Sun, Chiron will stay about 8 years (because Aries is a massive constellation). But when it moves within Saturn's orbit, into the sign Libra, it takes less than 11/2 years to speed through the sign.

This will help you plot where the comet is and when:

http://www.astro.com/swisseph/swepha_e.htm

Chiron's influence in Libra is the most hurried, and events in the world related to this transit occur sometimes at breakneck speed. Therefore then, its first square comes somewhere between you being 6-23, (just to reiterate it is easy to find when yours was, just not for me to do it as a sweeping statement for everyone). This is when it has moved 90 degrees around your chart.

It goes into opposition at 180 degrees and again, depending on how it is travelling this can happen between 13-30 years old. The second square will be between 35 - 46 and then it returns around your 51st birthday.

So, when I was born in '71, Chiron was in Aries (he's in Pisces now as I write). Aries being the baby of the horoscope (first sign) is all about the self too, about satisfaction of overcoming any obstacles that get in the way of self-fulfilment. (It is interesting that that's where he spends the most time and so we must suspect that is where he likes it best.)

What we'll do now is look at each house in turn and there are two things to see here. The first is which part of the body the house rules. This is not necessarily related to Chiron per se, it is just the rulership of each house. That said it can give you insights into which part of the body Chiron might affect as it moves around the natal chart. (That will be easier to understand when you see my "case history" in the first house.

Next we also talk about what "the psychological burden" tends to be depending on which house Chiron was in at the moment you were born. It is certainly a weird prediction that we can see what the problems of the child may be from where Chiron is at the time of the birth but it does seem to pan out that way.

Natal first house

Ruled by Aries (It is such a big constellation and thus so many areas are covered so it does not have a planet as such. If it did though, it would be Mars): (Find out more about Mars medicine in Sweet Basil Book)

Body parts covered:

The head, nose, blood (in particular the arteries) the muscles and sinews.

(So we'll do this house like a case history because it is my house. Please don't look at me. This is terrifying opening this wound. I feel entirely vulnerable but hey ho…let's rip the plaster off.

Those of us with Chiron in the first suffer crippling self-doubt and a total lack of self-worth. We often feel we have no right to exist or to assert ourselves. We worry that we might get "found out" for being not the person that we present to the world. There is an amusing question that people ask me at job interviews that always makes me smile. "If I asked your past colleagues about you, what would they say?" and it makes me laugh because they always think they are really clever to ask it and most of the other interviewers seem to have read the same book, but I always answer frankly "They'd say Liz is lovely until you get to know her." This is true. They do. And on one level that makes me feel quite secure that I am not too predictable and can be really ruthless when I need to be, but on another level I feel like they may have seen the real darkness inside of me which I would not want anyone to see. A part of me that I really despise. A part I feel is fundamentally unacceptable. I was shocked to find this awareness of the dark place and its unacceptability is symptomatic of people born with Chiron in the first house.

So we as a collective set of First House self haters have developed a coping mechanism, a kind of mask, that stops the world looking too closely at who we are, for fear of being found out. We over compensate and as you go through the houses you will see this over compensation as a theme. Because of the wound, we create a diversionary tactic. People with Chiron in the first, either become people pleasers and always put others first, or we become totally self-involved in our own problems. Many of my closest readers might have an epiphany about me here because people often ask me for tons and tons of help that

I will happily give then somehow I switch off and I am sure people wonder what the hell they did to deserve that. (In fact, I know they do because I have lost several friends doing it!) In actuality, they did nothing, I simply became overwhelmed by my own problem and could not cope with anyone else's for a while.

Often we find it hard to stand up for ourselves or to find the courage to ask for what we want. Consequently, we self-sabotage in an outrageous way looking for people to pay us some attention to divert us from the utter hatred we have for ourselves inside. We think that if they can love us, then perhaps there maybe something worth loving? We create situations that force people to reassure us that we are. Not only do we have this ridiculous self-sabotage mechanism (which incidentally my mum lives in fear of with me because I have a habit of ripping my life entirely to pieces to escape the pain) but we are often frustrated with life and have this underlying rage that we turn inwards.

But on the other side of the coin we are inveterate martyrs. We refuse to let anyone help us in return. We are profoundly self-sufficient to the point of being prone repeatedly to burnout. In truth we don't do everything ourselves because we know that we can it is because we are profoundly ashamed that we may not be able to.

Often people who are born with Chiron in the first may have had a difficult or traumatic birth. On one hand that makes absolutely no sense to me since that means that for eight years (whilst Chiron was moving through Aries) there were no good births but on another it really resonates. My mum always talks of how a "Big Black nurse held you under a tap" and you started to cry and she reckoned that until I was about thirty I never had a happy day. And truth be told, I was a miserable kid!

Many have trouble initiating actions or projects or the compensators, like me, rush into doing things, or hesitate because they doubt themselves or feel insecure.

A very important trait to observe here, is we first housers also have a very useful arrow to shoot that gets us out of things very well. We *become ill in order to avoid making important decisions*, facing difficult issues or to prevent us from taking actions that might alter our status quo.

Often we feel feel ugly or deformed. Many are ashamed or embarrassed by their bodies. We all feel awkward and uncoordinated and most of us actually are (You try walking with two human legs and two hooves, see how far you get!)

In her video on Youtube, Jean Wiley speak of how, when she sees the charts of my fellow housemates she sees someone who doesn't feel safe in life; they don't feel viable. Often on investigation she has found that the mother has not wanted to have the child and there has been a deep psychological imprint of the psyche of the child in vitro, and one would presume it was also very easy for the child to perceive how wanted it was once it came into the world. (Although I have to say this was not true for me, or if it was it has been well hidden.)

Physically, since this is my "case history" did you notice the physical attributes of the first house?

We have established I have Chiron as my rising planet at three degrees and so therefore in my first house. What happened to me to force me out of recruitment into writing and eventually into writing about healing? I got a blood clot in my lungs! It is *really* weird isn't it?! Mum also freaked me out by pointing out that I have always had some kind of unexplainable pain and discomfort in my left leg that I attribute to Restless Leg Syndrome*! No, I refuse to imagine that it's not a weird Chiron arrow, mum. I don't like that thought at all!*

Natal second house

Ruled by Venus (Find out more in depth in Rose book)

Body parts are:

*Throat, palate lips, neck, **ears**, cheeks, chin, thymus, thyroid*

This house seems to pertain to strange associations with financial resources and material goods. That they seem to feel that their power comes from manipulation of resources. Whatever they do for people, they expect there is something that has to be returned. Consequently, their perception of fairness may be very different to mine for example. You might find this person comes from a very wealthy background but there was always a very exacting standard to achieve to be worthy of a handout. Conversely, of course, they may have come from a very poor background, where there was a suspicion of people who had money.

So here we might see problems with people being very jealous and possessive leading to these self-sabotaging behaviours we have seen. On the other side of the coin, they might see any kind of wealth or possessions as an encumbrance and the last thing they want to do is tie themselves to that. Consequently, these people have a very strange relationship with money. They may spend, spend, spend or they will do whatever it takes to keep it far, far away from themselves.

Strangely often these people perceive their body as a resource too, and see it as wounded, tainted or unreliable. They have a relentless anxiety that it might let them down and here is very much a basis for somatic illness.

Trust is really a watchword for these people and remember how we talked about the Sun medicine allowing us to trust our creativity and allow it to flow. These people really need this. They don't trust their bodies, they don't trust their creativity or their ability to manifest and they certainly don't trust anyone around them. You may hear them talking about "Everyone being out for themselves...."

You will certainly see these people struggling to bring abundance into their lives and likewise they will seem to bring illness into themselves too. The Sun is shaded in their outlook and they seem to be magnets for money problems, turbulence and health issues.

One of the primary reasons these people do so poorly in life is they are unable to let things wash over them. They take things extremely literally and then they really allow themselves to get drawn into situations. They are unable to just see people's remarks as "their own stuff" and they feel it must be about them. This can often bring about quite a spiral of problems.

Natal Third House
Ruled by Mercury (Find out more in depth in clary sage and monarda books)

Brain and nervous system, shoulder mantle, arms, hands

Here the wound is with the mind or with learning. Often it speaks of a rather negative experience of school or of siblings who were cruel and perhaps teased. It could also be that the sibling had been ill and so took all of the attention away. For whatever reason they will feel that they were not heard and there will be a real wound with the sibling relationship that is probably ongoing.

You will definitely recognise throat chakra issues here: difficulty expressing yourself and being heard by others. You might see physical manifestations of people who literally cannot express themselves, so perhaps they stutter or likewise you might see stress related asthma. Breathing problems is definitely a big one.

Look at a chart of a dyslexic and it would not be shocking to see Chiron in the third. Foggy thinking and confusion especially if a person becomes overwhelmed by too much information.

With third house people there is a lack of balance between rational thought and intuition. They are either far too rational so there is no intuition of any kind or on the other extreme they are completely off with the faeries. They kind of give up on thinking and traverse life entirely through feeling. The first set of people seem to be exactly those Battaglia conveys when he says of Helichrysum: "*may help to ground people who have lost contact with the earth, and become too cerebral*"

These people can have extremely destructive or negative thought patterns for their main part, because they will not talk about what is going on in their head. They have tremendous difficulty expressing their feelings, or putting them into words and so consequently avoid any kind of emotionally charged subjects of conversation.

Natal Fourth House

Ruled by the moon (Find out more in depth in clary sage book)

Rules glandular tissue so the breasts, ovaries, testes, uterus, stomach (although I am going to say tummy here as in the bit that gets fatter, the outer fleshy tissue).

This wound seems to have something to do with the root family values and its association with receiving love, to do with mothering and their need for security. Often these people will feel like their sadness is like a bottomless pit that no amount of love can fill. Perhaps we might see that they had a very confining home environment or conversely that they were cast out. Perhaps there was a reason that the mother was dependant on the child, if she was disabled, for example.

It seems to be fairly easy to identify a fourth house person because they are very intense and brooding and really their own personal disturbance is quite unsettling to others around them. Would they be dressed in Emo togs? I don't know, but they will have a frown on their face!

Contra to their frightening outward appearance these are really compassionate people. They can intrinsically sense when someone is hurting. These people know pain because they have lived it intimately. They really resonate with compassion. Barbara Hand Clow describes how she often sees clients who have not yet learned how to transmute this energy into a way of healing others yet and these people tend to exhibit neurological problems such as Epstein- Barr (Precursor to Mono/glandular fever), Candida albacans or shingles.

(Here we can see how a plant that is anti-microbial, anti-fungal specifically against candida and is reputed to be able to help the herpes simplex might come in useful!!!)

Natal Fifth House
Ruled by the Sun so this is very important here

Heart, circulation, the back (in particular the upper back) the eyes and the spleen.

This is a weird place because Chiron is about learning through experience and so is the fifth house so consequently its effects are doubled. Then add to it that it is ruled by the Sun and you can really see how the effects may increase exponentially.

The fifth house pertains to the inner child and the ability to play, to be spontaneous and carefree.

We might see this wound come from being brought up in a very restricting home environment where it was not encouraged to play, create or build. This dynamic often leads to real feelings of inadequacy and so we can see this in patterns of acting out where someone dearly wants to be the star of the show and then lunges into black despair of feeling like a failure if something goes wrong.

These people can often go through life feeling frustrated and resentful that it is never their turn to shine, that they have never been given the opportunity or that the people around then do not recognise their talents.

This play dynamic is also very important in the case of addictions and how Chiron often brings about an over compensation. This house also rules quick relationships and children as well as recreational sex. Here we see odd relationships with sexuality where it is poles apart from being something attributed to love. John F Kennedy had Chiron in the fifth and it was only after his death that his sexual behaviour patterns came to light. Often there will be murky behaviour or these people will set up experiences for other people that will teach them what they want to know. I'd be interested to find out where it falls in EL James's chart or even, if he were real, in Christian Grey's!

Natal Sixth House

Also ruled by Mercury (Find out more in depth in clary sage and monarda books)

Bowels, intestines, alimentary system, respiratory system

Often this has to do with upsets and not feeling secure in one's day to day living. This is where we are going to expect to see the hypochondriacs and it is probably comforting for them to see that there is something "wrong" with them after all. These people have sensed a lack of wholeness for a very long time. There has been something amiss that the doctor has not been able to identify or fix and yet it still lingered there.

These people are very astute and have strong relationships between their emotional and physical bodies. Often though, whilst there is a sense that something is working against them they worry incessantly about it but don't actually do anything. This might be because they are sick of drawing blanks from the doctor, of course.

They have an innate lack of trust for their bodies and so by extension of themselves. Often you will see these people shying away from taking on responsibility in life or at work because they do not trust their capacity to fulfil their obligations (What if they get ill?).

This group of people are utterly preoccupied by themselves and their ailments. Their way to compensate is routine. This might mean they have unbelievably rigid dietary or exercise programmes (for fear of getting ill). They are obsessed by their routine and are very inflexible about work. Consequently, it is quite difficult to order their lives.

Conversely, there are those who cannot organise their lives because their illness is ruling it. They have very little structure and the chaos around them seems almost symptomatic of their emotional and physical state.

What's wonderful about these people though, is they really can help other people to organise their lives. They are very used to charting their possible ups and downs and plotting how they can cope around them and this is fantastic medicine for those who are sinking under the chaos of well....chaos really!

Here you might want to read the Monarda book because that looks carefully at mercury's affinity with lists and collation. It is a very interesting dynamic.

Natal Seventh House

Ruled by Venus (Find out more in depth in Rose book)

Kidneys, digestive system

Often this speaks of relationship issues. Perhaps the parent was absent or missing from the child's life for any number of reasons. It can be divorce, parent way in the military or in prison or even that there was not enough money to go round and so the child was put up for adoption. The possibilities are endless of course, but what this sets up very real concerns about relationships always going wrong. That the person is kind of toxic to relationships. And this can become a self-perpetuating prophesy as the person acts out repeating patterns that only serve to destroy their relationships.

Often the person has many blame issues, they project their fears and insecurities onto people around them. They will mirror what they see as bad behaviour back at partners and will become very, very defensive in their outlook.

After a while relationships tend to go out of the window because this set of people simply think "not going there". There is too much pain for them. They keep being abandoned. They keep being rejected. They keep being hurt.

Consequently, the pattern is often to sabotage until they come to conclusion that there is no-one out there for them.

Natal Eighth House

Ruled by Pluto (Find out more in depth in Vetiver book)

Reproductive system, in particular the genitals

Here the wound seems to be with dependency. Perhaps the child felt there was no-ne to lean on, no-one to turn to and that they were utterly alone in the world. It might have been because a parent or grandparent died, I suppose. Likewise, it might have been because mum was otherwise engaged with a new baby, because the eighth house is to do with birth and death.

This perceived "abandonment" leads to issues about dependency. So there may be a manipulation of controlling others so they cannot leave them. Deeper, it might manifest as this dreadful fear that someone could be taken from them at any time. They may become overly dependent on other people or conversely of course, refuse to depend on others and be everyone else's crutch. When that one falls apart I can imagine that could be extremely psychologically crippling.

Here too, we see problems to do with sexual separateness. That the person might continually feel sexually unfulfilled and yet be able to satisfy their partner's needs very easily. They do not have the innate understanding of two become one.

This seems reminiscent of the submissive wife toiling her sensuous garden in the Kama sutra building a lasting commemoration to unity with her yellow amaranth.

Natal Ninth House
Ruled by Jupiter (Find out more in depth in Holy Basil book)

Liver, pancreas, gall bladder, adrenals, feet, pleura

Ruled by Jupiter, the energy of wisdom and authority, when Chiron aspects this house it makes a person feel they have no authority, no wisdom or a lack of understanding of the philosophies of life. This often derives from the person's unease that they were inadequately schooled. Perhaps mum and dad did not believe "our kind" go to college, or their grades had not been good enough or they simply decided it was not the life path they wanted to follow but then went on to regret it.

These people are great students of life and tend to be advocates of lifelong learning seeking to compensate from this weakness in wisdom they perceive that they have.

In some cases, they can struggle to find meaning in anything and you might see these people will experience a bolt from the blue that radically changes their perception and their way of life. As a result, they take on the role of religious zealot and make long pilgrimages to Holy Shines or seek to understand other cultures and societies.

It might also be that these are children that were brought up in very religious households and they bear the wounds of their religion, so for example Catholicism and its relationship with sex being dirty.

In her video, Jean Wiley speaks of how she often seen this transit in people who have been in concentration camps and of course we should remember that these wounds that cannot be healed are very much to do with ancestral memory or our race and nationality and the pain that this imparts.

Natal Tenth House
Ruled by Saturn (Find out more in depth in Spikenard Book)

Skin, teeth bones, joints, depression,

Here the wound can be to do with reputation and authority. On the most mundane level, you might see that the person has difficulty in setting and achieving goals. They find it hard to find their societal niche and somehow are just not succeeding.

You find them in jobs that they have held for many years and are often suffering at the hands of a dreadful boss who abuses verbally or, in some cases, physically.

Often this will be a pattern that has come from a child realising that they have no interest in following the dreams that make them happy because it only irritates the parent. Consequently, the parents vicariously erase their failures through the successes of the child. And if the child does not live up to this expectation, well let's just say the parent is not very nice.

So here the person has no perception of their true worth because they are always being measured by someone else's standards and how good you make that other person look. People stay in these abusive jobs because they worry how it will look on their CV, moving so close to retirement etc.

Likewise, they can't see their own innate magic. They view themselves as worthless unless they can see as tangible reason why they are not. They work to the targets that other people set them to ensure they measure up in that person's eyes but usually cannot find the courage (or see a reason) to set their own.

"Trying" anything outside of their ordinary becomes something that they just don't do. They are scared to try to succeed because they fear the wrath of failure more. Worse they are scared to try because of the sting of ridicule they expect to come hurtling their way.

Natal Eleventh House
Ruled by Uranus

Nervous system, pituitary gland, nerves of the back including spinal cord and sciatic. In partnership with the Sun also rules circulation and the pulse.

I would also think of it for nerve pain, sciatica r neuralgia and would consider using it with rosemary.

These people probably really identify with the half man half horse with human legs because they really don't feel they fit in anywhere either. To a certain extent this is true because they inhabit their subconscious world far more than the rest of us would want to do.

It's like they have a telephone line directly into the collective unconscious and they feel the shifts of energy before they happen.

Are they weirdos? Well, yeah, kind of, they are because they are unsettling. They are very forward thinking and so by the time every one has caught up with whatever they had been trying to explain, the world has moved on and so are they.

They don't fit in with other people and because of that they tend to reject groups too. The problem is that actually what they would like more than anything is to have friendships and so they feel desperately lonely inside.

We're going to see peer group issues here. Probably quite rightly they are suspicious of the world. The chances are they also have experiences of being bullied.

The lesson for this group of people (See! In the end they did find a group...I'm all for a happily ever after) is to start to recognise that the world is not entirely full of nasty people, there are some quite nice ones too. As they start to see the Sunshine about this they often become a real champion of the supressed causes, a leader toward their issues of emancipation.

Natal Twelfth House
Ruled by Neptune

Pineal gland

These are the people who feel entirely at odds with themselves. Potentially they have been extremely tapped into other realms for many years but it is just not something that is accepted in their family, consequently it has been suppressed.

These people sense that they have a very deep secret that must be protected so they do not open up to anyone and keep themselves very private. For them the wound is being able to trust the gifts they have been given and to begin to accept themselves.

So why look at the houses?

I think this is a very interesting insight to gain, especially if the person seems to have no particular *reason* for their dis-ease. Things like fibromyalgia, IBS etc. with a somatic link but also I have a really strong sense of it being useful for people who can't get pregnant. Think of Artemis being the goddess of childbearing but never having been a mother of a child herself. Look at what Chiron would do if it aspects the eighth house. Here, although Helichrysum is tonic to the endocrine system (very helpful with fertility issues) here I suspect the medicine would be more about the dreadful pain this puts the couple through and helping them find a way to navigate their way through that to live a happy life without the blessing they so desperately crave. To me, this is just as important a medicine than the unlikely result of a sudden pregnancy.

In addition, I cannot help but think of that set of would-be parents who cannot manage to carry a pregnancy to term because the blood keeps on clotting and attacking the body (This is how my own blood clot happened in my lungs; I was pregnant at the time.) Those people who have Hughes Syndrome or Factor V Leiden – inherited conditions - how strange would it be if Helichrysum thinned the blood (which it does) and alleviated that challenge. Did you notice in the African medicine? There were several mentions of indications for ladies who had previously had troublesome pregnancies!

The interesting thing about these Chironic transits is, because of their very nature of falling under his rulership, and he is ruler of complementary medicine...they would **all likely respond better to complementary medicine** than to orthodox. Given that Helichrysum has an overall tonic action to the organism then we might suggest that Helichrysum might, more than often be the best essential oil to choose over any of the other...kind of like throwing a dart at the board and hoping that it will hit something. Whack some Helichrysum on and hope it finds the target!

Here we see a far more holistic medicine for the in/sub-fertile couple than just using nutmeg, say, to boost the pituitary or rose to tighten the womb. Will it help? Don't know. A drop of Helichrysum in a blend certainly wouldn't hurt here, would it?

Ok so let's quit floating in "what if" land, and see what happens if we use Helichrysum in the physical realms. First let's have a look at what the aromatic experts have to say and then we'll visit the labs and see if their ideas stack up.

Helichrysum Healing of the Physical Body with Aromatherapy

Skin

By far the most common assertion made by aromatherapists is that we use Helichrysum for skin care and that it will treat / alleviate scarring. Theophastrus suggested that if the herb were roasted with honey it would cure all burning and tearing of the skin. How does that suggestion compare with modern usage with essential oils?

One of the largest skin care companies in the world have selected immortelle as the main ingredient in their skin care range. The oil has anti-aging properties, gently preserving the skin and creating a more "everlasting" complexion. We'll see, in a moment, this is thanks to its anti-oxidant properties.

Scarring

In 1991 Dr Daniel Penoël explained that Helichrysum stimulates production and then protects new cells and that this is even true if the wound is deep and still bleeding. He refers to it as the "Super Arnica of aromatherapy"

This protection is very important and Kurt Schnaubelt elucidates upon it for us. He says "Components in Helichrysum italicum have been shown to mediate their tissue protective and regenerative quality by effectively scavenging free radicals. (Sala et al 2002)

ROS (reactive oxygen species) are generated by the organism but are generally *induced* by external factors. ROS are involved in arteriosclerosis, heart disease and aging. Secondary metabolites with conjugated double bonds (alternating single and double bonds, which allow electrons to be delocalised) such as Helichrysum, act as radical scavengers." In other words, they stop the cells from aging so quickly thereby promoting longevity.

Jeanne Rose defines how mixing it with rose hip oil will smooth and reduce scar tissue. (I won't cite it over and over but this mix of Helichrysum and rosehip seems to be the magical elixir that most people agree cannot be beaten)

Schnaubelt agrees. He states: "Helichrysum italicum works for all conditions in which inflamed tissue needs to be calmed down and regenerated."

He lists it for scars, whether they are from recent surgery or for older ones that a patient has had for a long time. He also recommends it for tissues which have become inflamed and to reduce hematoma. He would use it for allergic skin reactions, to ease the pressure of haemorrhoids, to break down keloid scar tissue and to smooth stretch marks. To ease the pain of inflammation of tendonitis.

Peter Holmes asserts that it has *skin regenerating, collagen stimulating and anti- inflammatory* actions.

An experiment in 2007 by Voinchet and Giraud-Robert testes *Helichrysum italicum var serotinum* blended into a maceration of musk rose on patients who had just undergone cosmetic and reconstructive surgeries. They wanted to assess the effects it would have on the inflammation of the skin and the bruising. Amazingly, when the usual length of hospitalisation, after these surgeries, would be twelve days, more than half of the patients were able to go home after just five. In all cases the post-operative scarring had been reduced.

They attributed the success of the oil to the italidones and they felt certain that the neryl acetate had contributed to the analgesic success. They identified that there seemed to be some anti-staphylococcal and antistreptococcal actions which they felt must have reduced infection. They felt that the musk rose had played a part in preventing keloid scars from developing,

In 2006 Rhiannon Harris recommended the possibility of using a Helichrysum *hydrosol* to treat slow to heal wounds associated with significant tissue trauma.

Suzanne Catty made an important point with her recommendation of using the hydrolat to reduce the inflammation on the skin after surgery, that the Helichrysum also helps to move the anaesthetic along from the liver.

She also recommends the floral water for in-growing hairs.

Burns

I think I would still go for lavender in the panic after a burn but Jeanne Rose disagrees. She says Helichrysum with rose geranium.

Acne

Palz writes "*Treating acne with Helichrysum in dilution has proven more effective than the use of any other essential oil.*"

I would suggest that it is not only the emollient and beauty aspect here, but when you get to the science you will be stunned just how many bugs and germies it can restrain. It will be the antimicrobial properties of the oil that are just as important here.

I would add that the anti-inflammatory nature of the oil makes it a good choice for rosacea. Here, I would use with gardenia oil and, actually, it might be interesting to see how effective the hydrolat would be here too.

Abscesses

Dex has a horrible one on his neck. No amount of antibiotic oils has shifted it. Likewise, the galbanum does not seem to be setting the world on fire but Helichrysum seems to be doing the job. Bizarrely, I have since found out that the correct name for an abscess that will not heal is...*chirotic.*

Eczema, Dermatitis and Psoriasis

The avenues where this can help are myriad. Firstly, of course, it helps to heal the skin. Underpinning this sort of illness is often non-fatty liver disease (See both my eczema and liver books) and so this hepatic boost is fundamental. But the emotional link of the language of the skin is all about feeling vulnerable about how people see you. It is an inherited disorder for many, so both of these seem to be Chironic issues.

Immortelle is emollient, smoothing the skin, softening it and making it less prone to breakages and splitting.

Anti-allergenic

For all of the reasons above, and simply because it is such a benign oil, blended with violet leaf, Helichrysum is like the softest cotton glove to sensitive skins.

Jennifer Rhind Pearce recommends it for allergic issues such as eczema, asthma and hay fever.

Peter Holmes suggests taking it internally to treat food allergies.

We'll address the internal issue in the safety section.

Radiation burns

Beautifully soothing to radiation burns after cancer treatment.

Inflammation

Building on the assertions of Dioscorides that it heals pains in the hips or, indeed, gout. Likewise, fractures, he says and internal and external divisions (I think we can fairly say we covered external in skin).

Its anti-inflammatory skills lend it to all kinds of joint discomfort, rheumatism and arthritis, tendonitis, bursitis, and any other kinds of RSI. I guess the other big gun for this would be frankincense.

I was a bit freaked out by Jeanne Rose's suggestions. She explains that she has found it most effective when blended with Sweet wormwood – (one of this weird plants that wavers on and off of hazardous oils lists) and Yarrow and other azulene-laden oils. Why did it freak me? Latin names? *Artemisia arborens* and *Achillea millefolium*. I feel sure the Greek gods are howling at laughter at me as I write!!!!

I think I would also be tempted to reach for some laurel if the pains seemed to be in the head and neck. There seems to be an association to me, with these Olympic crowns but also with problems with the second house astrologically.

Blood

Helichrysum is a very effective anti-coagulant.

Elaine Zimmermann was able to shine a light on the reason for this in her book *Aromatherapie fur Pflege un Heilberufe*. She explains that one of the active components in the oil is Beta-Diones, (also often listed as *italidones*). *"These components have anticoagulant properties, making [Helichrysum]also effective for the treatment of hematomas."*

Bruises

Jeanne Rose recounts the same as I have found with bruising. That, if you apply Helichrysum neat to the wound, the anti-hematic properties stop the blood accumulating and so a bruise just does not form. (Since I like to milk any wound I have got to get out of housework, I tend not do this...!)

Suzanne Catty agrees. She suggests adding the hydrosol makes the expensive essential oil go further when treating bruises.

Thrombosis

Price and Price build on this and say that because of the blood thinning action they would suggest it for red veins, haematoma, thrombosis and prevention of bruises.

As ever Gabriel Mojay's work touched me at the very deepest level. He speaks of the blood here in the likeness of Chinese medicine, as the life force of the body and spirit. "

"Everlasting oil's capacity to dissolve clots give it on a subtle level, the power to break through the deepest, most "stuck" of negative emotions and restore compassion not only for others but also for oneself".

Jade Shutes similarly communicates how Helichrysum helps to balance qi energy and the blood.

Phlebitis (Paltz 1984)

Coronary complaints (Paltz 1984)

Haemorrhoids

Varicose veins

Arterial Circulation (Hozzel)

Liver

J Paltz speaks extensively of Helichrysum in his work *Le fascinant pouvoir des huiles essential*" written in 1984 (I cannot be sure, but I wonder if this the oldest "aromatherapy" reference to it? I don't think I have found older.)

He speaks of how Helichrysum detoxifies the body of drugs and nicotine. We'll come back to this because other authorities also suggest it for addiction.

The oil is also considered to be a strong chelator, supporting liver function and potentially drawing heavy metals and toxins out of the body. Salvatore Battaglia tells us," It is well known as a stimulant to the liver, gall bladder, kidney, spleen and pancreas- the organs responsible for detoxifying the body".

Later you will see the science backs this up and that Helichrysum is protective of the liver.

Hepatitis

I found a lovely paper written by Dr Annmarie Giraud-Robert and some work she had done treating patients with Hepatitis. Sixty patients were treated in all, who were chronic carriers of either Hep B or C.

She had used a selection of ravintsara, Labrador tea, carrot seed, thyme ct thujanol, laurel, niaouli and Helichrysum to treat the group. Sometimes these might be used as monotherapies and also they were used as complementary to allopathic treatments (the doctor's meds!)

Those patients who had been given a dual therapy of oils and allopathic medicines made 100% improvement whereas those who had used only essential oils only saw a 64% improvement although there were two complete cures of Hep B in that group.

Digestive system

High blood sugar

High cholesterol levels because it is blood thinning (Hozzel)

Respiratory

Palz cites it for whooping cough and as being anti-viral. Valerie Worwood recommends Helichrysum for rebuilding a weakened immune system.

We cannot overlook how effective it is as a decongestant, so think of it for sinusitis, rhinitis or any kind of stuffiness or congestion. A couple of drops on your palms or on a handkerchief will do wonders to ease the pain. It seems likely that it is the heavy presence of terpenes in its composition that create this magic.

It is a very useful oil to use for bronchitis or asthma, because of its softening and relaxing effect. It relaxes the bronchial tubes and turns solidified catarrh into liquid. This tonic affect will be very helpful alongside frankincense and monarda, for instance.

J Palz recommends it for whooping cough.

Since the mouth is the entry to the upper respiratory tract, this seems as good a place as anywhere for the suggestion of using One teaspoon of Helichrysum hydrolat as a mouthwash. This would be wonderful as daily hygiene against gingivitis and inflamed gums but also the perfect salve against the trauma of having had a tooth extracted.

Genito Urinary

Dioscorides suggested that Helichrysum should be given in wine to people who were struggling to urinate.

I have found recommendations of it being used in traditional medicine for herpes and syphilis. I found science backing up herpes and HIV but not specifically syphilis yet. (Chances are though I might have found it in the African Helichrysum research if I had looked hard enough, because there probably isn't that much commercial incentive for the Western drug companies to research treatments for syphilis over diabetes, say.)

Reproductive

Promotes menstruation- Dioscorides.

Suzanne Catty imparts how she has used the hydrosol in combination with rock rose flower essence to treat endometriosis, fibroids and painful periods.

Hearing Problems

There seems to be a great deal of excitement from people who have been able to rid themselves of tinnitus and even improve their hearing with Helichrysum. Many have combined it with marjoram and are massaging up onto the bones around and behind the outer ear. Others are using it diluted with olive or sesame oils onto cotton balls that they are placing into the ear. The interesting thing about these testimonies is they seem to all be on hard of hearing forums and the conversations are between people who seem to know nothing else about aromatherapy. In some ways then we could see these "trials" as blind (as opposed to deaf!) and potentially more reliable in comparison to the myriad essential oils' sales pages.

The Emotional Healing of Helichrysum

I suppose we could analyse the anti-depressant quality of Immortelle as being *strengthening* too. Certainly, it seems to be like a no-messing physio that says "you have to do this!" There is certainly a sense of "You are not getting away with this. It's happening. Deal with it." I don't think it really builds courage as such, or even determination, more resilience and patience. You do what you have to do. I agree with Worwood when she says that it encourages calm, acceptance, patience and perseverance.

I would heartily recommend you read Dr Bruce Berkowsky's monograph on Helichrysum. If you are not familiar with his work, he aligns essential oils against other healing modalities like crystals and homeopathic treatments to gain an insight into the "phytoessence" of the healing. I love his work. I could have listed so many more of his insights but a) they are his b) the book would have gone off in too many directions. Nevertheless, I regard every word he writes as gospel!!!

He lists the emotions indicated for Helichrysum as:

shock; fear; phobias; debility; lethargy; nervous exhaustion; nervousness; anxiety; insomnia; depression; moodiness; resentment; anger; bitterness; emotional repression; emotional denial; problems with inner identity; rigidity; deeply-ingrained negativity; difficulty incarnating spiritually.

(Buy his article on Helichrysum here: http://naturalhealthscience.com/spiritual-phytoessencing-medica.php#!/Helichrysum-Materia-medica/p/46534256/category=8817235)

Ixchel Susan Leigh, in Aromatic Alchemy, agrees with what Gabriel Mojay described about Helichrysum's affinity with compassion. She says it promotes longevity, enhances intuition, creativity and feelings of compassion. Kathy Padecky tells us it promotes calmness, inner strength and perseverance, awareness and acceptance.

Peter Holmes distinguishes it as being the primary oil for trauma care (emotional and physical). He describes it as nurturing, calming, harmonizing and grounding. He explains that Helichrysum will "*reduce apprehension, irritability and mental unrest and that it helps untangle emotional knots and resolve past emotional trauma*".

When I read Margaret Ann Lembo's work about Helichrysum it reminded me of the African usage of the incense to strengthen new babies. She elucidates that it is used for anointing during ceremonies of entry and exiting this planet. The African incenses and the funeral wreaths. It made me smile.

She conveys how it "disincarnates entities to help them to find their way to the light or to the other side". (That must be the di-ketones too. Dr Malte Hozzel describes ketones as being the disincarnators of the plant kingdom...)

She beautifully illustrates the Chironic perspective when she says that Helichrysum "improves the overall outlook, helping you transcend every challenge". She advises "Be aware of how well you treat yourself and beware of inner chatter."

Dr. Hozzel of Oshadhi outlines how all of this is achieved when Helichrysum is able to "*stimulate the right side of the brain, supporting development of intuition and creativity and contributing to the relaxing and healing dynamics of deeply rooted emotions, stress like anger and resentment. Therefore, it is a fantastic help to PTSD*" He recommends diffusing for 45 mins.

Joy and Cynthia at Stillpoint reminded me of the nature of the plant, how it even grows through rocks and how, even though it is gentle, it is very powerful. I like their recommendation that it adds an "added punch" to other oils in a blend.

Of every description of the oil, and there are many because it seems to encourage people to wax lyrical, somehow, I love Patricia Davis's description that it is "honey for the psyche". She describes how it can activate our intuitive brain and helps us in visualisation, meditation and in creative endeavour.

Magickal Uses:

It is said that if Helichrysum grows around your home or gateways it will keep cats away from your property. Many cultures grow it bring longevity and healing into the home. Helichrysum is reputed to help with scrying and channelling practices. (I hear the Croatian chemotype is better for this than the Corsican and I have certainly found that it speaks its wisdom very clearly. I have found several rituals where burning the leaves are said to invoke the spirits of the departed. I love what StarChild have written on their website about it: "its everlasting nature can teach us about the immortal nature of the soul and the mysteries of self-regeneration."

Astute, I feel. Very, very astute.

Clinical Evidence of *Helichrysum italicum*

Wounds that do not heal...

When I started this book, I thought that might only apply to **skin** and **abscesses.** How wrong could I be? What a long way we have come. Now, I am about take you deeper into this strange paradigm.

- To the **herpes simplex**
- To **HIV**
- To the heinous **multidrug resistant infection** that strikes the fear of God into warzone hospitals - ***Acinetobacter baumannii***

And to many other illnesses that seemingly have no hope of healing.

But then, bizarrely, they respond unusually to Helichrysum....

As previously discussed there are species aplenty to choose from to research and actually I could have gone on for months because Helichrysum is a fascinating species but for the purpose of the book I am going to try to stay as close as possible to the commercially available essential oil *Helichrysum italicum*. There are other commercially available chemotypes of Helichrysum but with the diversity of this one subspecies being complicated enough...well, we would have to be heroes to attempt that frankly, and we are but yet mere mortals, are we not?

Also, I'd like to stress, at this point, that virtually none of the medical research in this book has come from experiments using essential oils, most are ethanoic extractions. This means that the data may not completely cross over to the essential oils because the active component may not be able to pass through distillation and thus may not be found in the essential oil. That being said, I will be reaching for my bottle more and more, I think.

There was a report published in 2014 in the Journal of Ethnopharmacology by the Health Sciences Research Centre from the *Universitat of Beira Interior* in Portugal has made my job extremely easy here because they did a very thorough study of all the available studies in the clinical databases made into *Helichrysum italicum.*

They explain that usage of the plant has been very well documented throughout Italy, Spain, Portugal, Bosnia and Herzegovina.

Traditionally the flowers and leaves are used to treat allergies, colds, coughs, skin, liver and gall bladder conditions, inflammation, infection and sleeplessness.

When the clinical trials have been assessed, it seems to be the flavonoids and terpenoids that are so effective against bacteria in particular staph aureus. Let's start here:

Tissue

If this book shows us nothing else, it is that there are always more things at play than a person could ever hope to perceive.

The problem lies underneath the skin, insidiously attacking the person within. We see that in the research here most of all.

You and I would use Helichrysum to heal the skin in the hope that no scar will form. But what of those wounds that remain open. What of the people who have to lie in hospital beds for months upon end, perhaps in comas, perhaps not, but have to be turned to avoid bed sores?

Imagine if a sore were to form.

We all know how dangerous a hospital becomes then. Perhaps that patient might have been safer in Chiron's cave away from the contagions that lurk on the toilets and damp surfaces of the wards.

Perchance, their wounds maybe septic from shrapnel, or the hospitals out in the field are simply not well enough equipped for the time and resources needed to tend to whole units wrecked with one terrifying bomb.

What then?

Well sadly, a whole new set of bacteria have evolved to exploit these very situations.

Anti-microbial

May 2009, and researchers in Marseille from the Université de la Mediteranée found that *Helichrysum italicum* significantly reduced multidrug resistance to a number of bacterial pathogens. *Enterobacter aerogenes, E-coli, Pseudomonas aeruginosa, Acinetobacter baumannii.*

Enterobacter infections can take any number of forms. Blood infections, any kind of lower respiratory tract infections, infections in the skin and soft-tissue, urinary tract infections (UTIs), endocarditis, intra-abdominal infections, infections of the central nervous system, and eye infections. It is one of the primary risks to the success of lung transplants, for example, entering the system and compromising the body's ability to heal.

Pseudomonas is a gram negative infection that can affect virtually any systcm, and will mainly be found in patients that have been hospitalised for over a week.

It might present as affecting the respiratory tract in cases like pneumonia. It can affect the blood and attack the heart in conditions such as endocarditis.

Likewise, it can affect the ear or the eyes, urinary tract, gastro intestinal tract, the bones or joints or the skin. Terrifyingly it can also affect the brain causing brain abscess or meningitis. All of this from one single bacterium.

Acinetobacter baumannii is a particularly unpleasant fiend and one that makes me think of Artemis's sacred plant the most. In his paper "*The emergence of a successful pathogen*" A.V. Peleg of Beth Israel Deaconess Medical Centre and

Harvard Medical School describes the germ's predilection for patients lying helpless in intensive care wards and it largely responsible for people having to stay there for so much longer.

It has been found in hospitals for many decades but is now a particular difficulty to *military* hospitals. Its evolution seemed to gather pace during the Iraq War with more and more injured soldiers being attacked by this horrible bacteria, gaining it the new moniker "Iraqibacter".

There is only one conventional treatment that *baumannii* has not evolved to conquer, but this is a very toxic antibiotic with many side effects and as such, is not the most desirable medicine. Consequently, scientists are searching fast for other medicines that may be able to overcome the Iraqibacter and in a petri dish...Helichrysum can. (The test was with an extract, not with the essential oil so we can still only speculate how effective it would be.) So what is the active constituent that had helped to protect Chiron's heroes after they had been wounded by hydras and gorgons? What is it, in the oil, that Artemis uses to keep her battle field virgins safe? It is ***geraniol***, the scientists can now tell us.

Oral bacteria

Back in the aromatherapy section, there were mentions of using Immortelle as a mouthwash. In 2004 the Università di

Messina, found that Helichrysum was also effective at inhibiting the oral pathogen Streptococcus mutans.

Inflammation

To me, this is the most exciting section so get yourself a cup of tea before you begin to read it because I promise you, you'll be thinking of the ramifications of it for hours.

When the oil was analysed it was found that H. italicum, its components (acetophenones, flavonoids and phloroglucinols) exerted an inhibitory action in several inflammatory pathways and mediators including the metabolism of arachidonic acid.

Very interesting, I am sure. But what on Earth is arachidonic acid?

Hold onto your horses, ladies. This is about to get interesting.

Arachidonic acid is a fatty acid found in large amounts in the brain and other parts of the body. Neurological health is fundamentally dependant on there being sufficient levels of this acid because it helps to maintain the cell membrane fluidity of the hippocampus and protects it from oxidative stress. Disturbed metabolism of arachidonic acid is seen in Alzheimer's and bi-polar disorder. Arachidonic acid activates a syntaxin protein involved in growth and repair of neurons.

Cool, thank you.

Still don’t understand...!

Well, let’s just revise what the hippocampus is responsible for.

It is essentially involved in the formation of memories and then acts as a shipping centre to send them to the long term memory which it does when we are asleep. More importantly for us, as aromatherapists, and in the context of this book, it is the part of the limbic system that allocates a sensation or emotion to a memory.

In other words, if you smell a particular oil and it reminds you of something horrible and your stomach lurches...that’s the hippocampus at play!

Actually there are two hippocampi, one on the right of the brain, one on the left and they are the shape of sea horses (Hippo means horse – in fact the Latin name for Sea Horse is Hippocampus hippocampus!). The left hand one is involved in verbal memory, so you remember names etc., the right is thought to be more concerned with spatial memory in terms of location (I remember where the chair is in the room.)

You might remember we spoke about this spatial memory in the clary sage book, because we discussed at length about how it can be affected in Alzheimer’s Disease. Scientists are now starting to uncover that different parts of it do slightly different things, and so react to different aspects of learning. For example, a 2003 study showed that all the concentration and learning involved in navigating the complex maze of the capital's street had caused the rear section of London cabbies hippocampus to grow!

I noticed that the Portuguese report had said that Helichrysum was used for sleeplessness and it is not an oil I would have suggested for that. Add to that Dioscorides and Artemedorus's comments about how it makes you dream, and this makes this even more interesting because studies show that the hippocampal activity during sleep after training or any kind of learning leads to better memory of the lesson the next day. Somehow it helps you to assimilate the data better. I wonder then what we will find Helichrysum can do, in the future for the veterans who keep reliving the same nightmare night after night.

Incidentally, there might be some confusion here that the memory stays in the hippocampus. It doesn't it stays there for the short term and then it is shipped off and filed as long term memory in the hypothalamus. Sleep is absolutely critical in this process.

So that's interesting isn't it? And I keep recalling the statue of Chiron and Achilles from Corinth (http://www.whatischemistry.unina.it/martachille.jpg) and how rapt the boy seems listening to his lesson.

Helichrysum presents the degradation of arachidonic acid, and protects the new acid as it is produced.

Research has also show that supplementation of the acid, if given early in life, actually leads to increased intelligence and, if continued this improved intelligence continues to grow.

Bu there is more, because arachidonic acid, if you remember it is not only found in the brain, it is also found in the body. *Arachidonic acid* is marketed as a body building supplement. It increases lean mass, strength and anaerobic power in experienced body builders. Other clinical trials showed that supplementation of arachidonic acid lead to anaerobic capacity and performance.

Remember how the kama sutra discussed using it to enlarge the lingham...? Guess where else there is arachidonic acid...yup, you got it. It wasn't the buffalo milk. People, if you like your man hung like a stallion (or at least half man, half horse) then Helichrysum may be able to help.

(It brings a whole new dimension to the phrase "make hay while the sun shines", doesn't it?!)

What's more, supplementation of arachidonic acid (in broiler chickens) was also able to significantly able to raise low sperm levels to register as normal ones. The Africans are absolutely right to use Helichrysum for virility.

Remember the hoplites, chiselled and gleaming in the Sunshine...Who knows, perhaps it was the Helichrysum that kept those torsos looking so damn fine!

https://www.ncbi.nlm.nih.gov/pubmed/12559384

Actually, more specifically we know that it is 1 (4-hydroxy-3-(3-methyl-2-butenyl) which is the acetophenone in Helichrysum that stops the arachidonic acid from metabolising. This was ascertained in 2003 and became a basis for research into novel anti-inflammatory and analgesic drugs.
https://www.ncbi.nlm.nih.gov/pubmed/12559384

(Incidentally, if any of you want to supplement more with arachidonic acid it is found in omega 6 oils fish and is metabolised from linoleic acid. There is absolutely no science to support this thought, but I think I would go carrier oils with GLA including borage and evening primrose so there was more source of linoleic acid to synthesize from.)

Oh just as an aside, on the subject of the kama sutra, David Crow of Floracopaeia says he has seen evidence of Helichrysum promoting hair growth too.

Anti-fungal

You may have noticed that I have a love of anything old. The older the better, and whilst I have been researching this book I have been to a number of museums looking at Roman and Ancient Greek artefacts. It makes my heart sing to see something old can last for all these years. Imagine my pleasure then, to find a paper by the *Institute of Botany and Botanical Gardens in Belgrade* to investigate the usage of *Helichrysum italicum* **essential oil** as an antifungal to protect ancient cultural artefacts.

The primary components of the oil they used were γ-curcumene (22.45%), α-pinene (15.91 %) and neryl acetate (7.85 %). *H. italicum* essential oil had a moderate antifungal effect against fungi they had collected from the cultural heritage objects. The most susceptible fungi to their treatment were *Epicoccum nigrum* and *Penicillium* species, while the most resistant was Trichoderma viride. The *H. italicum* essential oil was also inhibiting to *Aspergillus niger*. (Without going way of track, you might also remember *Aspergillus* was the bad guy that triggers so many people's coughing fits in the bronchitis book.)

Antifungal oils are interesting because, actually there are not many natural anti-fungals in existence. The next trial is useful because it involves man's best friend, his dog.

Malasezzia

Malassezzia pachydermatitis is a fungal infection that affects dogs. Normally the conventional treatment would be using a therapy called Ketaconazole taken 10 mg/kg a day along with chlorhexidine at 2%

This trial by the University of Pisa, from September 2014, compares the results of 10 animals treated with the conventional treatment versus a new essential oils concoction called Malacalm. Bravely, they published their recipe!

- *Citrus auriantum 1%*
- *Lavandula officinalis 1%*
- *Origanum vulgare 0.5%*
- *Origanum majorana 0.5%*
- *Mentha piperita 0.5%*
- *Helichrysum italicum 0.5%*
- *Carrier or almond and coconut oil*

Twenty animals had their treatment applied to their skins twice daily for a month.

At the end of the treatment both groups had improved significantly with no adverse effects. After 180 days a follow up appointment was performed. The dogs which had been treated with the conventional treatment were beginning to show recurrent symptoms of rashes and scratching but the essential oils group had none.

They found that the ingredient that inhibited in the lowest dilution was, predictably, the oregano, super herb, that it is. It was effective at just 0.8% There had had to be a lot of Helichrysum before it did its job ...10% dilution, Peppermint had kicked in at 1%, marjoram at 1.3% and neroli/ Petitgrain/orange (not clear which) at 2%.

Candida

The acetophenones, phloroglucinols and terpinolals are anti-fungal against candida albacans (Again, I would suggest you cross reference this with the candida section in my eczema book reader. This has a massive part to play in treating skin conditions and allergies).

Arzanol

This is a phloroglucinol extracted from Helichrysum italicum. It has been found to be anti-inflammatory, anti-HIV and antioxidant.

It has been found to affect how the T Cells replicate in HIV. The function of T Cells, (also known as T Helper cells or sometimes CD4s) is to protect the body against infection. They send signals to activate the body's response if they encounter an "invader" this might be infection or a bacterium.

HIV destroys the entire immune system by killing these T Cells. It replicates the clever mechanism of the T Cell, encouraging it to multiply and then spreading the infection throughout the body.

In a petri dish, *Helichrysum italicum* has been seen to prevent this replication. HIV drugs cannot cure the disease, but they can help make the patient's life longer, and help them to live a healthier life.

Helps them to live with the wound that cannot be healed.

Arzanol also affects the release of IL1 β, IL6, TL8, and TNF-α, all of which are inflammatory markers and which it is proven are triggered and exacerbated by stress and hostility.

Strangely, South Africa is home to over 35 different species of the Helichrysum genus and of 30 that have been trialled five of the species have been found to be anti -HIV. Strange of course, because the ground has offered up a medicine in Africa where it is thought the disease derived from. http://www.sciencedirect.com/science/article/pii/S0367326X15000891

Herpes

In 2003 it was also found that the flavonoids in Helichrysum italicum inhibited HSV. To you and I, that is the Herpes Simplex Virus.

Because Arzanol has such a diversity of mechanisms it provides great hope for treating auto-immune disease and also cancer.

Liver

Many internet pages say that Helichrysum removes chelates from the liver. I cannot find evidence to support this statement, although I don't doubt for a second it exists.

I did find evidence that it is used in phytoremediation, a term you may remember from the vetiver book, in that it can remove toxins and heavy metals from the soil. In particular it removes zinc and so I would suspect it would do the same for the liver too.

I also found a fascinating trial that proved that Helichrysum *protects* the liver.

Digestion

In December 2013 the University of Navarra in Spain looked at how Helichrysum and grapefruit affected the blood sugar after eating.

The Helichrysum had the greatest inhibitory activity of α glucosidase an enzyme located in the brush border of the small intestine. If you take oral anti-diabetic drugs these are also α glucosidase inhibitors. The function of the enzyme is to prevent the digestion of carbohydrates such as starches and carbohydrates so they can be absorbed into the small intestine.

Helichrysum was found to be better at inhibiting than α-amylase (another enzyme) whereas grapefruit was not quite as good but was equally as effective as α- amylase. Helichrysum then, inhibits the enzyme making the digestion of the sugar far more effective and healthy.

Now, can I have a round of applause please for our friends the micc plcasc. Thcy havc lingcrcd long behind the curtains in this book. Come on rodents it is your turn in the spotlight (I have missed them, have you?)

In 2015, Navarra University built on their findings about grapefruit and Helichrysum using some thirty-eight Wistar white rats. After days of normal eating, they were separated into groups f no supplementation, grapefruit supplementation and Helichrysum supplementation. Fed the same, the grapefruit and Helichrysum rats gained less weight over a five-week period, had lower blood serum levels of insulin and liver TBARS (lipid peroxidation)

The report concludes: Helichrysum and grapefruit extracts might be used as complement hypocaloric diets in weight loss treatment. Both extracts helped to reduce weight gain, hyperinsulinemia, and IR, improved inflammation markers, and decreased the HFS diet-induced oxidative stress in insulin-resistant rats.

https://www.ncbi.nlm.nih.gov/pubmed/25599391

Intestinal Spasm

The Journal of Ethnopharmacology published a paper in Dec 2013 written by the Department of Pharmacy in Naples supports the use of traditional usage of Helichrysum tea for intestinal complaints and spasms.

They had isolated a mouse ileum, in an organ bath, then stimulated it into spasm with acetylcholine and barium chloride. When the Helichrysum was added to the bath the spasm was reduced.

Tiliroside

Tiliroside is a flavonoid isolated from Helichrysum italicum which has been found to be anti-inflammatory, anti-microbial, anti-oxidant and anti-tumour.

Insect repellent

The two-spotted mite, *Tetranychus urticae Koch* is an annoying insect that damages crops especially fruit and vegetables. There are conventional pesticides developed but the bug has evolved and become pretty much resistant to the treatments

A treatment was developed using a mix of five extracts: [i.e., *Allium sativum L. Rhododendron luteum S. Helichrysum arenarium L. Veratrum album L. and Tanacetum parthenium L.* . The mix achieved a 10% mortality on the pests but sadly did not affect the eggs.

In November 2010 *The Department of Tree Sciences* from the Università di Pisa tested Helichrysum against the mosquito *Aedes albopictus*. This is a hard creature to manage because most pesticides have to be added to the water where the mozzies congregate. Adding chemicals to water obviously brings about its own set of health concerns. Yarrow, Helichrysum and lavender all brought about a mortality rate of between 98.3-100% of the drugs. Helichrysum was able to bring this about with a dilution of just 1.8%

Blood

When I was at Botanica this year, Madeleine Kerkhof Knapp Hayes gave a wonderful lecture on CO2 extraction and its comparisons with essential oils. It was the talk of the conference with everyone deliberating whether these differently extracted plant extracts might become a whole new, perhaps even more important, aspect of aromatherapy than essential oils. The reason is that, as well as being a very pure form of extraction, it is also able to pull far more of the molecules (and in larger quantities) across from the plant into the extract. (Boswellic acid is found within the frankincense CO2).

I was intrigued by this and when I started the research for this book, I found a paper discussing that ***scopoletin*** could be found in far higher quantities in the CO2. Indeed, when I checked Tisserand and Young 2013 list of constituents, its seems not to be found at all within their analysed essential oils (or perhaps it is in such small quanities it does not show). Yet in the Co2, the researchers from Croatia, Bosnia and Herzegovina had found it contained molecules 1.933mg / 100%.

Scopoletin is interesting to them because is a very important constituent for regulating blood pressure. Not only can it lower BP, but it can push it up when the person's blood pressure is too low too. It has a *balancing* action.

It is also bactericidal and exhibits very strong reduction effects on E-Coli, Staph aureus as well as other staph species. It inhibits *Kliebsella pneumonia* and *Pseudomona aeruginosa.* It exhibits an anti-inflammatory effect especially in the lungs so it is very useful for people with asthmatic or bronchial conditions.

Excitingly it also regulates serotonin so effectively helps sufferers of anxiety and depression. Here is your Sunshine, people!

Using Helichrysum in your treatments

Look at the amaranth, on tall mountains it grows, On the very stones and rocks, And places inaccessible.

Popular Greek Song

Blending

Base Note

Blends well with

Blends well with - Bergamot, Chamomile, Clary Sage, Lavender, Geranium, Rose, Rosewood, Myrrh, Frankincense and spikenard, Rose, Lime, Neroli, Orange, Petit Grain, Sage and Ylang-Ylang Oil amongst many others

It is a sweet, thick fragrance with honey like notes and a slightly liquorice note. Very sexy!

Safety Data

Undiluted Usage

I can hear the safety mob screaming and vying for my blood already, but I am merely citing the experts here. (It weren't me guv, it's the other fella!)

Dr Schnaubelt asserts that using neat on an open wound would be the most effective and safest avenue because it avoids complications from adding other fatty oils into an open sore

Ingestion

Again here, he says "One drop of essential oil in a glass of water will restart liver activity after a "Crise de fois". (That'll be Prometheus's vulture then...would anything less traumatic count as a liver crisis then? Yes of course, read my Essential Oil Liver Cleanse to see that liver toxicity is insidious. That being said, I think don't do this too often.)

As I stated earlier Peter Holmes suggests that ingestion may be indicated for conditions of tissue re-generating, especially where there has been some hyper permeability of the gut and acute and chronic inflammations

As long as I was happy about the source of the oil, then I would consider taking Helichrysum internally in times of crisis. Of course, drinking the hydrolat may be preferable to ingesting the essential oil. Suzanne Catty suggests that would be the perfect thing to do after a prolonged illness.

Recommended Dilution

Tisserand and Young 2013 recommends a standard dilution of 0.5% because there have been very rare and mild skin irritations reported.

Martin Watt says to use it in 4% dilution max and that seems a better recommendation to me. I will confess to having used it extensively, neat, whilst I have been writing the book and have seen no adverse effects, only very fast healing.

Drug Interactions

Tisserand and Young 2013 offers no recommendations about drug interactions but I came across a paper that makes me feel otherwise.

"Reversible inhibition of three important human liver cytochrome p450 enzymes by Tiliroside."

https://www.ncbi.nlm.nih.gov/pubmed/21031626

This paper says there may be possible interactions with drugs with substrates of CYP3A4, CYP2C9 and CYP2C8

This is not an area I feel confident commenting on so for explanations and deeper data: http://www.pharmacytimes.com/publications/issue/2008/2008-09/2008-09-8687

Please take these to your physician for advice on whether your drug will be acceptable with use of *Helichrysum italicum*.

Alfentanil (Alfenta)	Ixabepilone (Ixempra)

Alfuzosin (Uroxatral)
Almotriptan (Axert)
Alprazolam (Xanax)
Amiodarone (Cordarone)
Amlodipine (Norvasc)
Aprepitant (Emend)
Atazanavir (Reyataz)
Atorvastatin (Lipitor)
Bepridil (Vascor)
Bexarotene (Targretin)
Bosentan (Tracleer)
Bromocriptine (Parlodel)
Budesonide (Entocort)
Buprenorphine (Subutex)
Bupropion (Zyban, Wellbutrin, Voxra)
Carbamazepine (eg, Tegretol)
Cevimeline (Evoxac)
Cilostazol (Pletal)
Cisapride (Propulsid)
Clarithromycin (Biaxin)
Clonazepam (Klonopin)
Clopidogrel (Plavix)
Colchicine
Cyclophosphamide (Cytoxan)

Ketoconazole (Nizoral)
Lapatinib (Tykerb)
Levomethadyl (Orlaam)
Loperamide (Imodium)
Lopinavir (Kaletra)
Loratadine (Claritin)
Lovastatin (Mevacor)
Maraviroc (Selzentry)
Mefloquine (Lariam)
Methylprednisolone
Midazolam (Versed)
Mifepristone (Mifeprex)
Modafinil (Provigil)
Nefazodone
Nevirapine (Viramune)
Nicardipine (Cardene)
Nifedipine (Adalat)
Nimodipine (Nimotop)
Nisoldipine (Sular)
Nitrendipine (Baypress)
Oxybutynin (Ditropan)
Oxycodone (Percodan)

Cyclosporine (Neoral)
Dapsone (Avlosulfon)
Darunavir (Prezista)
Dasatinib (Sprycel)
Delavirdine (Rescriptor)
Dexamethasone (Decadron)
Dihydroergotamine
Diltiazem (Cardizem)
Disopyramide (Norpace)
Docetaxel (Taxotere)
Donepezil (Aricept)
Doxorubicin (Adriamycin)
Droperidol
Dutasteride (Avodart)
Ebastine (Kestine)
Efavirenz (Sustiva)
Eletriptan (Relpax)
Eplerenone (Inspra)
Ergotamine (Ergomar)
Erlotinib (Tarceva)
Erythromycin
Estazolam (ProSom)
Eszopiclone (Lunesta)
Ethinyl Estradiol
Ethosuximide (Zarontin)
Paclitaxel (Taxol)
Paricalcitol (Zemplar)
Pimozide (Orap)
Pioglitazone
Praziquantel (Biltricide)
Prednisolone
Prednisone
Propoxyphene (Darvon)
Quazepam (Doral)
Quetiapine (Seroquel)
Quinacrine
Quinidine
Quinine
Ranolazine (Ranexa)
Repaglinide (Prandin)
Rifabutin (Rimactane)
Ritonavir (Norvir)
Saquinavir (Invirase)
Sibutramine (Meridia)
Sildenafil (Viagra)
Simvastatin (Zocor)
Sirolimus (Rapamune)
Solifenacin (Vesicare)

Etoposide (Vepesid)
Exemestane (Aromasin)
Felodipine (Plendil)
Fentanyl (Sublimaze)
Finasteride (Proscar)
Flurazepam (Dalmane)
Fosamprenavir (Lexiva)
Galantamine (Reminyl)
Gefitinib (Iressa)
Granisetron (Kytril)
Halofantrine (Halfan)
Ifosfamide (Ifex)
Imatinib (Gleevec)
Indinavir (Crixivan)
Irinotecan (Camptosar)
Isradipine (DynaCirc)
Itraconazole (Sporanox)
Sufentanil (Sufenta)
Sunitinib (Sutent)
Tacrolimus (Prograf)
Tadalafil (Cialis)
Tamoxifen (Nolvadex)
Tamsulosin (Flomax)
Teniposide (Vumon)
Testosterone
Tiagabine (Gabitril)
Tinidazole (Tindamax)
Tipranavir (Aptivus)
Topiramate (Topamax)
Triazolam (Halcion)
Vardenafil (Levitra)
Verapamil (Calan)
Vinblastine (Velbane)
Vincristine (Oncovin)
Ziprasidone (Geodon)
Zolpidem (Ambien)
Zonisamide (Zonegran)
Zopiclone (Imovane)

The Musical Vibration of Helichrysum

The Croatian Helichrysum vibrates in E minor (also known as G Major) o, which is one sharp in the key signature. I had imagined that the Corsican would vibrate around a similar note but when I compared it, it vibrates closer to C. Nevertheless, that becomes too complicated so we'll stick with the Croatian as our anchor here.

If you do not have a musical repertoire in your head, imagine some kind of classical guitar music. Most classical guitar is written or improvised in the key of E minor because it is very natural finger placement for the chords.

I'm going to start off back at Artemis's Amaranthia and some thoughts about those beautiful youths all dancing, full of potential, before the sacrifices of the sheep. It really made me think of another bitter trade that was about to be made. It made me think of the guilt of the people who knew that had to send them out to their deaths. Lastly, Sting sees the same correlation between this feeling of betrayal and the need for some kind of substance to escape the interminable reminder of it.

Children's Crusade:
https://www.youtube.com/watch?v=88WOPnJBKiA leads to addiction

Usually I would start off the music a bit more lightly but there is no escaping pain with this book. It stands at its very core. Where Bergamot and Mellissa are uplifting, Helichrysum has a different job to do. It says I cannot take your pain away from you but I would love to help you bear it.

So switch the Sun off for a moment. Let's take Helichrysum out of the equation. Let's steel ourselves again for a reminder what these tired angry minds might be feeling. Let's hear what this paradox might look like, so that we can understand what we have to work with when we add our italicum into the mix. Perhaps there is a smile on the face, but let's seek out what the internal dialogue really sounds like.

Wrong side of heaven (You heard this earlier, so feel free to skip it if you can remember it.)

https://www.youtube.com/watch?v=o_l4Ab5FRwM

Zombies: The Cranberries

Another head hangs lowly

Child is slowly taken

And if violence causes the silence

Who are we mistaking

But you see it's not me

It's not my family

In your head in your head

They are fighting

With their tanks and their bombs

And their bombs and their guns

In your head in your head they are crying

https://www.youtube.com/watch?v=6Ejga4kJUts

The theme of the song is, of course, the Northern Ireland troubles which I saw first-hand because I married the son of a Belfast minister. We would often go across to Ireland to see his family who lived very close to the Falls Road and often we could hear echoes of problems as we dropped off to sleep. We would see tales of the atrocities when we were at home in England but when we travelled back across the water, the TV seemed to run nothing else. I was young and found it futile and troubling. I am proud to say that several of my in-laws played an active part in the peace process. I was always an outsider. I did not share their blood line and ancestry and could not understand the collective nuances of the fight. This song illustrates clearly how the battle seemed to have no beginning and no end and how it always seemed to be “the others” who were at fault.

And then we have this strange (Sun-) golden woman on the cross surrounded by Greek youths with bows who eventually sacrifice themselves on the cross. Honestly guys, this time the synaesthesia (hearing the musical note of the essential oil) seriously freaked me out!

Have you got your bottle of Helichrysum at the ready? Let’s sprinkle a couple of drops into our patient’s cream.

Let’s hear the whisper of the song....

There never was a more beautiful demonstration of the difference between what people say from what they actually feel, than the enigmatic lyrics coming up on the screen. It takes a moment or two for you to realise there has been a divergence and what you are actually seeing in people’s silent thoughts of pain. A most appropriate sense of Helichrysum’s Sunshine secret whisper of “*when you’re sure you’ve had enough, hang on*”.

Everybody hurts:

https://www.youtube.com/watch?v=ijZRCIrTgQc

I'd be failing in my job if I did not ask Evanescence to sing us My Immortal, their song about the wounds that will not heal. She starts off very much in the vein of our Chironic heroes hidden from the sun:

"*I'm so tired of being here....*"

And how the memories of the past keep on haunting her.

https://www.youtube.com/watch?v=5anLPw0Efmo

Amy Grant has the honour of turning Helichrysum's story around. Her bewitching melody sings the moment when Helichrysum begins to break the rock hard defences and convinces the patient that, probably, it might be OK to take a look at the Hell they have been avoiding and to risk feeling their pain. https://www.youtube.com/watch?v=6WnAia_QRIo

Here comes the Sun : The Beatles

https://www.youtube.com/watch?v=bgiQD56eWDk

Now I have to credit beliefnet.com with the next video because not only did I laugh all the way though his blog post about Chiron because it was so astute and witty, but he also found the very best representation of Chiron's lesson.

Ladies and Gentlemen, please allow me the honour of introducing you to...Peg Leg Bates

https://www.youtube.com/watch?v=hayM4B7hcBQ

Wasn't he wonderful?

I wanted to say goodbye on a hopeful note, because this book is raw and quite frankly, a bit depressing, isn't it? I'll send you on a way with a reminder that Chiron's lessons are always hopeful. Unappetising, granted. But in the end, they're welcome, because they serve to deepen our human experience and lead us to a far deeper understanding of ourselves and what we are capable of. And so when Helichrysum is added into a blend, his Sunshine Medicine casts a glow to light thc gloom in the cave. If you are really lucky you might even catch a glimpse of Artemis lifting her bow and aiming for something you cannot even perceive. What is it? Perhaps something hidden beneath the skin, deep, where only the gods might know.

As the arrow, dipped in Helichrysum, strikes a point of hidden pain, unseen the most profound healing can begin.

And when it does...when the Sun streams in...

Well these folks,

These are good times.

The Good Times; Chic

https://www.youtube.com/watch?v=eKl6EZShaaw

So congratulations for making it this far and thank you. I shall reward you with one of the most beautiful pieces of music I have ever heard. Truly, only you and I could ever understand why on Earth this song could be about Helichrysum. First Elton John's so you can get the lyrics and then the maestro because it would be wrong not to.

Treat your medicine well. Go out into the world. Heal.

And Live like Horses.

https://www.youtube.com/watch?v=kAa51oYSI8U

https://www.youtube.com/watch?v=zw_gEpGqnqQ

The Rose and the Amaranth

A Rose and an Amaranth blossomed side by side in a garden, and the Amaranth said to her neighbour, "How I envy you your beauty and your sweet scent! No wonder you are such a universal favourite." But the Rose replied with a shade of sadness in her voice, "Ah, my dear friend, I bloom but for a time: my petals soon wither and fall, and then I die. But your flowers never fade, even if they are cut; for they are everlasting."

Aesop

Conclusion

I wonder what you will make of my little book?

Many of you will want to order a wrap of whatever drug I have been ingesting I am sure! I'd love it if you could leave me a review and let me know. These really make a difference to whether I sell more books or not!

I am not sure how I feel about it myself. I am very calm, given that I am typing this, two days before I have to despatch it to get to the NAHA conference in NAHA and that is unusual for me. I have not been in the slightest bit stressed and I have simply plodded on knowing I will make the deadline and I amazed to find I have. Not only that, but I keep laughing at everything! I really am as daft as I was at 15, and it feels great!

I have discovered a great many things about myself through my studies into Chiron and I have to say understanding these things has made me be a bit gentler on myself. I now find I amuse myself rather than irritate or upset. That is really quite the liberation for me.

I have also found that Helichrysum and sleep do not mix for me. I do sleep, but my goodness, Dioscorides was right, I really do dream. While that has helped me write the book, discovering many truths and deep corners that in daylight I wound rather ignore...to be honest I left those bits of the cave dusty for a reason and I shall avoid this deep introspection for a while. It was a bit too acute for my liking...but then I have been snorting it in large amounts, bathing in it and goodness knows what!

It has definitely made the Sun come out though and you may be interested to know that Helichrysum cannot even grow in the shade. I like to think how the rays must be captured and held in the very lifeform of the plant until we strange humans decide to bottle it. Bottling it is most certainly a clever thing to do, I think.

I have enjoyed comparing the light and shade aspects of Chiron's medicine through Helichrysum and it has made me think a great deal about the psychology of military leaders and how they come to terms with thc dccisions thcy makc. Arguably the most famous son of Immortelle's famous isle of Corsica was the celebrated military leader Napoleon. After rising through the ranks of the army, eventually he reached the position of Emperor and was beloved of all his countrymen. But how the mighty fell, and very soon he was exiled to Elba (where Helichrysum also grows). Legend has it that Napoleon described how he could smell the Helichrysum long before he reached his homeland of the Macquis. The thought weighs heavy with me that perhaps, had he lived today Napoleon would have been remembered in a very different way. Scholars even go as far as to suggest it would be more accurate to remember him as a war criminal in studies today, because they think it was he who first created the gas chambers. I smile at the notion that a plant may have affected both his judgement and ours! Has it wafted its Sunshine grace over his history for us to see him so positively, I wonder?

Who can tell?

Chiron also rules synchronicity and I have to say these past few months I have been seeing coincidences everywhere. Not least that whilst I have been writing about a comet that rules complementary medicine, our species managed to land a satellite on another comet so we could see, not only what it actually looked like, but also possibly the origins of life on our own planet. One creation story standing right next to those of the myths of the Ancient Greek gods. It has felt very strange yet very connected.

Oh by the way...

I found something out from Gardener's World this morning- the genus name *Asteraceae* means *Star*...

What must be said though is my planetary rulership is hypothesis and speculation, nothing more. Just as there is no way to understand how a birthdate might affect the experiences of our childhood and then scar us for the rest of our lives, all I can say is this feels right to me. You must make your own interpretations as you feel fit. Perhaps in the end a question mark is more satisfactory than an ill-defined answer in the end anyway! Life is full of mystery and that's just the way I like it!

I have dedicated this book to Misty who is one of my students. She has worked so hard and fired dozens of questions at me. T begin with they were about dilution but recently the tone has changed and she is starting to look beneath the physical aspects of disease. I just wanted to tell her how proud I am of how far she has come. Hopefully this book will help her to make some treatments that can really help her beautiful family.

Before I go, I must say thank you to all of you who sent me supportive messages in the days after our friend Sam's crash and pledged money to her fundraising page. I am overjoyed to tell you that all your prayers have created what the British press and the medics are calling a miracle, with an almost complete recovery after just eight weeks. (For complete transparency, even though her story inspired this book the doctors have not wanted to use any oils or anything un-prescribed on her delicate skin grafts thus far, so I cannot take any of the credit. All the miraculous healing is all entirely down to the doctors, nurses and paramedics, down to Sam, her very courageous family and the support she has had from friends.) If you have not kept up with her story, you can find my daughter's best friend here:

http://www.dailymail.co.uk/news/article-3814394/Student-22-left-coma-horror-car-crash-saved-wiggled-toe-moments-doctors-turn-life-support-machine.html

I am so proud of Sam, my Aimée and her girlfriend Ola. They conducted themselves far more maturely in their support than I ever could have done, I think. Sam still has a great deal of rehab to do and will need a lot of care and new equipment. If you feel you could spare a couple of dollars we would be very grateful. You can find her fundraising page here:

https://www.gofundme.com/2uvxye7w?viewupdates=1&utm_source=internal&utm_medium=email&utm_content=cta_button&utm_campaign=upd_n

With that I am going to leave you, but please do stay in touch. I have busy days ahead speaking at the NAHA conference and then off to Shanghai to teach about skin care. Who knows what questions I shall bring back from there?!

Take very good care of you and speak soon, I hope.

Bye (and buy!)

Liz

PS the details of my course are on the next page, with notes on my other books. Oh and don't forget to leave me that review please!

PPS I got my Croatian Helichrysum from http://www.essentialoilscroatia.com/

Learn from The Secret Healer

If you fancy a bit more tuition you can take Elizabeth's introduction to aromatherapy. 93 videos about the fundamentals of aromatherapy and in depth information on 15 different oils.

Find the course at:

https://beta.ofcourse.co.uk/course/aromatherapy-essential-oils-advanced

Normally priced at £199, please use discount code **TEACHER_ELIZA82** to get it for £35 (around $50) as a little thank you for all your support.

About The Author

Elizabeth Ashley is an international speaker for the International Federation of Aromatherapists and the UK Director for the National Association of Holistic Aromatherapists. She is a prolific writer of professional articles, in particular for the IFA magazine Aromatherapy Thymes, Aromatika.hu, NAHA Journal and Holistic Therapist She qualified as an aromatherapist in 1993, and then passed her Advanced Aromatherapy Diploma in 1994. She has been practicing aromatherapy for almost 25 years.

In 1999, she fell into a whole new career in the aggressive commercial sector of recruitment consultancy. There she discovered her father's second hand car salesman genes had passed along and found she had quite a gift of the gab! More than that, she discovered she could sell...and then some.

In 2008, Elizabeth fell ill during pregnancy with a blood clot in her lungs. The pulmonary embolism prevented her from working and she started to write. Very quickly she gained her first contract as a ghost writer...a recipe book for cheese cakes!

In 2010 she was published professionally for her work on Galbanum - (*Ferula Galbaniflua*) oil in the Aromatherapy Thymes, journal of the International Federation of Aromatherapists, and on Tuberose – (*Polianthes tuberosa*)

oil by the New Zealand Register of Holistic Therapist.

In 2011 she was seconded on a consultative basis to Walsall Independent Treatment Centre, designed to be a rainbow bridge between traditional and complementary medicines. There she became aware of the rumblings of change in healthcare. Her book Sales Strategies for Gentle Souls explains the connotations of this.

Many of her books are aimed at helping qualified aromatherapists to expand their healing repertoire and build their businesses. She also writes for people who have an interest in essential oils and want to learn how to heal. Her in depth essential oil profiles chart the healing properties of plants from the most arcane depths of historic folklore up to the scientific lab trials of today.

She lives in Shropshire with her husband and youngest son, kept company by their Staffordshire Bull Terrier, Bella, and many shoals of tropical fish! Her elder son and daughter have graduated from university this year and make her prouder than anything ever could. Elizabeth Ashley is The Secret Healer.

□

Other Books by the Author

Why not check out my reviews?

75 Quick and Easy Aromatherapy Christmas Gifts Ideas: Essential Oil Recipes for Handmade Personalised Gifts

50 Easy Essential Oil Recipes for Skin Care Products for Dry Skin - Make Your Own Anti-Aging Moisturizers & Night Creams Professional Aromatherapy Skin Care Tips and Beauty Secrets

The Secret Healer Oils Profiles:

Some of the oils we have covered in this book will be familiar, but possibly not all. You may find some of the oils profiles deepen your knowledge and fascination for the art of aromatherapy.

Vetiver - (*Vetiveria zizanoides*): The Oil of Tranquillity

Monarda: *(Monarda fistulosa)* A Native American Medicine

Holy Basil: *(Ocimum santum)* An Ayurvedic Medicine

Rose - (*Rosa damascena*): Goddess Medicine; A Timeless Elixir

Sweet Basil - *(Ocimum basilicum)*– The Oil of Empowerment

Clary Sage- *Salvia sclarea*; Natural Estrogen? Alleviate Symptoms of Menopause, Premenstrual Syndrome and Period Pains. Reduce Muscle Cramps and Restless Leg Syndrome. Ease Depression Symptoms and Improve Memory and Cognition with Clary Sage

Spikenard -A Woman Anoints Jesus's feet -: Did She Use the Spikenard of Aromatherapy? *Nardostachys jatamansi* - An Essential Oil and Medicinal Plant for digestive problems, nervous disorders, anxiety, insomnia, epilepsy, seizures and fear

The Secret Healing Manuals:

Book 1 - The Complete Guide to

Clinical Aromatherapy & Essential Oils for the Physical Body

Download for FREE

Book 2 Essential Oils for Mind Body Spirit

The Holistic Medicine of Clinical Aromatherapy

Book 3 The Essential Oil Liver Cleanse

The Professional Aromatherapist's Liver Detox

Book 4 The Professional Stress Solution

Essential Oils and Holistic Health Stress Management Techniques for The Professional Aromatherapist

Book 5 The Aromatherapy Eczema Treatment

Healing Eczema, Itchy Skin Rashes and Atopic Dermatitis with Essential Oils and Holistic Medicine

Book 6 The Aromatherapy Bronchitis Treatment

Support the Respiratory System with Essential Oils and Holistic Medicine for COPD, Emphysema, Acute and Chronic Bronchitis Symptoms

Sales Strategies for Gentle Souls; Targeted Sales Training for Professional Aromatherapists

□

References

al, L. J. (2006). *Chemical composition, antimicrobial activities and odor descriptions of some essential oils with characteristic floral-rosy scent and of their principal aroma compounds* . Retrieved from Research Signpost: http://www.holzer-group.at/download.asp?id=372

al, S. M. (2013, 08). *Genetic and metabolite diversity of Sardinian populations of Helichrysum italicum.* Retrieved from Directory of Open Access Journals: https://doaj.org/article/4d9ee2b2fc164f86b18e7840a207fb07

Amaranth. (n.d.). Retrieved from https://en.wikipedia.org/wiki/Amaranth

Amaranth. (2012, 02 20). Retrieved from Dreams Nest: http://dreamsnest.com/amaranth/

Amaranthus (mythology. (n.d.). Retrieved from Myths of The World Wiki: http://mythworld.wikia.com/wiki/Amaranthus_(mythology)

Anand aromatherapy. (n.d.). *Helichrysum Essential Oil.* Retrieved from Anand Aromatherapy: http://www.anandaapothecary.com/aromatherapy-essential-oils/helichrysum-essential-oil.html

Angel Fire. (1779). *Chiron in the Natal Chart.* Retrieved from http://www.angelfire.com/journal/GregoryJdeMontfort/Chiron.htm

Angioni A1, B. A. (2003, 02). *Chemical composition, plant genetic differences, and antifungal activity of the essential oil of Helichrysum italicum G. Don ssp. microphyllum (Willd) Nym.* Retrieved from Pubmed: https://www.ncbi.nlm.nih.gov/pubmed/12568568

Antunes Viegas D1, P.-d.-O. A.-d.-O.-d.-O. (2014). *Helichrysum italicum: from traditional use to scientific data.* Retrieved from Pubmed: https://www.ncbi.nlm.nih.gov/pubmed/?term=helichrysum+italicum+herpes

Appendino G1, O. M. (2003, 04). *Arzanol, an anti-inflammatory and anti-HIV-1 phloroglucinol alpha-Pyrone from Helichrysum italicum ssp. microphyllum.* Retrieved from Pubmed: https://www.ncbi.nlm.nih.gov/pubmed/17315926

Arachidonic Acid. (n.d.). Retrieved from https://en.wikipedia.org/wiki/Arachidonic_acid

Aromed Aromatherapy. (Post 2014). *Helichrysum (Corsica)* . Retrieved from Aromed Aromatherapy: http://aromedofvt.com/products/helichrysum-corsica

Axe, D. (n.d.). *Helichrysum Essential Oil: Uses, Benefits & DIY Recipes.* Retrieved from What is Helichrysum Essential Oil?: https://draxe.com/helichrysum-essential-oil/

Battaglia, S. (2002). *The Complete Guide to Aromatherapy.*

Battistini, M. (2007). *Astrology, Magic, and Alchemy in Art.* Getty Publications,.

Baumann, H. (1993). *Greek wild flowers and plant lore in ancient Greece.* Herbert Press.

Bentley, R. (1842). *The History of the Manners and Customs of Ancient Greece,.* London.

Berkowsky, D. B. (n.d.). *Helichrysum* . Retrieved from Natural Health Science: http://naturalhealthscience.com/spiritual-phytoessencing-medica.php#!/Helichrysum-Materia-medica/p/46534256/category=8817235

Bianchini A1, S. F. (2009, 07). *Partitioning the relative contributions of inorganic plant composition and soil characteristics to the quality of Helichrysum italicum subsp. italicum (Roth) G. Don fil. essential oil.* Retrieved from Pubmed: https://www.ncbi.nlm.nih.gov/pubmed/19623548

Bigovic D1, B. S. (2010, 05 09). *Relaxant effect of the ethanol extract of Helichrysum plicatum (Asteraceae) on isolated rat ileum contractions.* Retrieved from Pubmed: https://www.ncbi.nlm.nih.gov/pubmed/20657488

Bizimana, N. (n.d.). *Traditional Veterinary Practice in Africa.*

Blair, K. (2014). *The Wild Wisdom of Weeds: 13 Essential Plants for Human Survival.* Chelsea Green Publishing.

Bradley, M. (2014). *Smell and the Ancient Senses.* Routledge,.

Brewer, E. C. (2001). *Wordsworth Dictionary of Phrase and Fable.* Wordsworth Editions,.

Buchmann, S. (2016). *The Reason for Flowers: Their History, Culture, Biology, and How They Change Our Lives.* Simon and Schuster.

Buckle, J. (2014). *Clinical Aromatherapy: Essential Oils in Practice.* Elsevier Health Sciences.

Cafe Astrology. (2002-2016). *Chiron in the Houses of the Natal Chart.* Retrieved from https://cafeastrology.com/articles/chironinhouses.html

Cappers, R. T. (2007). *Fields of Change: Progress in African Archaeobotany.* Barkhuis, .

Carrion, C. P. (n.d.). *Helichrysum italicum (Immortelle) Essential Oil.* Retrieved from http://thearomablog.com/helichrysum-italicum-immortelle-essential-oil-therapeutic-benefits/

Chinou IB, R. V. (96, 08). *Chemical and biological studies on two Helichrysum species of Greek origin.* Retrieved from Pubmed: https://www.ncbi.nlm.nih.gov/pubmed/8792676

Clarke, M. (2005, 2016). *Helichrysum, Corsican* . Retrieved from Nature's Gift: https://www.naturesgift.com/product/helichrysum-traditional-2ml/

Clow, B. H. (1987). *Chiron: Rainbow Bridge Between the Inner and Outer Planets.* Llewellyn Worldwide.

Conneely, M. (2012, 05 30). *Chiron, the Wounded Healer in the Birth Chart.* Retrieved from http://blog.starwheelastrology.com/chiron-the-wounded-healer-in-the-birth-chart/

Costea, M., & Tardiff, F. J. (2003, 07). *The Name of Amaranth - Histories and Meanings.* Retrieved from JStor: http://www.jstor.org/stable/41968150?seq=1#page_scan_tab_contents

Currie, M. (n.d.). *chiron-unappetizing-but-highly-nourishing.* Retrieved from http://www.beliefnet.com/columnists/ohmystars/2014/02/chiron-unappetizing-but-highly-nourishing.html

D'Abrosca B1, B. E. (2013, 11). *Spectroscopic identification and anti-biofilm properties of polar metabolites from the medicinal plant Helichrysum italicum against Pseudomonas aeruginosa.* Retrieved from Pubmed: https://www.ncbi.nlm.nih.gov/pubmed/24094434

Daughter of Chiron. (n.d.). *Artemis.* Retrieved from https://daughterofchiron.wordpress.com/2014/10/04/%CE%B1%CF%81%CF%84%CE%B5%CE%BC%CE%B9%CF%82artemisdiana/

Davidson, J. (15, 05 13). *Chiron In The Houses.* Retrieved from Stealing Fire From The Gogs : https://stealingfirefromthegods.wordpress.com/2015/05/13/natal-chiron-in-3rd-house/

Davis, P. (2012). *Astrological Aromatherapy.* Random House .

de la Garza AL1, 2. E. (2015, 08). *Helichrysum and Grapefruit Extracts Boost Weight Loss in Overweight Rats Reducing Inflammation.* Retrieved from Pubmed: https://www.ncbi.nlm.nih.gov/pubmed/25599391

de la Garza AL1, E. U. (2013, 12). *Helichrysum and grapefruit extracts inhibit carbohydrate digestion and absorption, improving postprandial glucose levels and hyperinsulinemia in rats.* Retrieved from Pubmed: https://www.ncbi.nlm.nih.gov/pubmed/24261475

Deiss, J. J. (1989). *Herculaneum, Italy's Buried Treasure.* Getty Publications, .

Dunphy, R. (2016, 01 19). *Essential Ol potlight - Helichrysum- Immortelle-Everlastin.* Retrieved from raedunphy: http://www.raedunphy.ca/blog/essential-oil-spotlight-helichrysum-immortelleeverlasting/

Eisdon, D. (2000). *Vibrational Healing: Revealing the Essence of Nature Through Aromatherapy* . Frog Books.

essential-oil-profile-helichrysum. (2014, 11 10). Retrieved from Cheryls Herbs: https://www.cherylsherbs.com/home/essential-oil-profile-helichrysum/

Farrar, L. (2016). *Gardens and Gardeners of the Ancient World: History, Myth and Archaeology*. Casemate Publishers, .

Folium Medica. (n.d.). *Helichrysum an Essential Oil With A History*. Retrieved from https://foliummedica.com/helichrysum-an-essential-oil-with-a-history/

Foti C1, G. S. (2013, 07). *Allergic contact dermatitis caused by Helichrysum italicum contained in an emollient cream*. Retrieved from Pubmed: https://www.ncbi.nlm.nih.gov/pubmed/23782363

Free Spirited Mind. (n.d.). *Chiron in the second House* . Retrieved from http://freespiritedmind.com/blog/chiron-in-the-2nd-house/

Grimaldi, P. (n.d.). *Astrology Online*. Retrieved from http://www.astrologyonline.eu/Graphic/Estrai_NewInt/Visual_Chiron.asp

Halil Erhan Eroğlu, c. a. (2009, 04 24). *Cytogenetic effects of nine Helichrysum taxa in human lymphocytes culture*. Retrieved from Pubmed: https://www.ncbi.nlm.nih.gov/pmc/articles/PMC2677150/

Harte, W. (1767). *The amaranth, or, Religious poems [by W. Harte].*

Hecker, J. F. (1838). *The Epidemics of the Middle Ages*. Haswell, Barrington, and Haswell.

Helichrysum. (n.d.). Retrieved from https://en.wikipedia.org/wiki/Helichrysum

Helichrysum Essential oil. (n.d.). Retrieved from http://www.edenbotanicals.com/helichrysum-croatia-organic.html

Helichrysum italicum From Corsica vs Helichrysums in General. (2006, 03 16). Retrieved from http://www.indiadivine.org/content/topic/1896068-helichrysum-italicum-from-corsica-vs-helichrysums-in-general/

Help with Hearing Challenges-Using Helichrysum EO. (n.d.). Retrieved from http://theresanoilforthat.blogspot.co.uk/2009/01/help-with-hearing-challenges-using.html

Herbs.info. (n.d.). *Helichrysum Essential Oil*. Retrieved from http://www.herbs-info.com/essential-oils/helichrysum-essential-oil.html

Heyman HM1, S. F. (2015, 06). *Identification of anti-HIV active dicaffeoylquinic- and tricaffeoylquinic acids in Helichrysum populifolium by NMR-based metabolomic guided fractionation*. Retrieved from Pubmed: https://www.ncbi.nlm.nih.gov/pubmed/25841639

In Search Of The World's Finest Helichrysum Essential Oil With Floracopeia's David Crow, L.Ac. (2016, 03 29). Retrieved from http://jihub.net/page/watch/vid2016ksh9iFxdEiI

Jasmine, B. (n.d.). *Natal Chiron Aspects.* Retrieved from http://www.aquarianage.org/west/planets/ch-nat02.html

Jokić S1, R. M. (2016, 09). *Supercritical Extraction of Scopoletin from Helichrysum italicum (Roth) G. Don Flowers.* Retrieved from Pubmed: https://www.ncbi.nlm.nih.gov/pubmed/27439115

Kabbar, J. G. (n.d.). *Chiron.* Retrieved from https://www.youtube.com/watch?v=fs8qdUFt-mk

Kladar NV1, A. G. (2015, 03). *Biochemical characterization of Helichrysum italicum (Roth) G.Don subsp. italicum (Asteraceae) from Montenegro: phytochemical screening, chemotaxonomy, and antioxidant properties.* Retrieved from Pubmed: https://www.ncbi.nlm.nih.gov/pubmed/25766915

Lawrence, B. (2013, November). *Progress in Essential Oils: Cinnamon Bark Oil and Extract, and Helichrysum Oil.* Retrieved from http://www.perfumerflavorist.com/fragrance/rawmaterials/natural/Progress-in-Essential-Oils-Cinnamon-bark-oil-helichrysum-oil-233507191.html

Lembo, M. A. (2016). *The Essential Guide to Aromatherapy and Vibrational Healing.* Llewellyn Worldwide,.

Leonardi M1, A. K. (2013, 03). *Essential-oil composition of Helichrysum italicum (ROTH) G.DON ssp. italicum from Elba Island (Tuscany, Italy).* Retrieved from Pubmed: https://www.ncbi.nlm.nih.gov/pubmed/23495152

Leyel, C. F. (2007). *Cinqfoil.* Health Research Books,.

Mancini E1, D. M. (2011, 09 08). *Chemical composition and possible in vitro phytotoxic activity of Helichrsyum italicum (Roth) Don ssp. italicum.* Retrieved from Pubmed: https://www.ncbi.nlm.nih.gov/pubmed/21904272

Mari A1, N. A. (2014, 08 05). *Identification and quantitative determination of the polar constituents in Helichrysum italicum flowers and derived food supplements.* Retrieved from Pubmed: https://www.ncbi.nlm.nih.gov/pubmed/24786189

Marina. (2016, 03). *Chiron the Planet Comet Asteroid.* Retrieved from http://darkstarastrology.com/chiron/

Marks, B. (n.d.). *Chiron.* Retrieved from http://www.bobmarksastrologer.com/chiron21.5.html

Martial, L. W. (2003). *Martial: Select Epigrams.* Cambridge University Pres.

Mastelić J1, P. O. (2008, 04). *Contribution to the analysis of the essential oil of Helichrysum italicum (Roth) G. Don. Determination of ester bonded acids and phenols.* Retrieved from Pubmes: https://www.ncbi.nlm.nih.gov/pubmed/18463581

Mastelić J1, P. O. (2008, 03). *Contribution to the analysis of the essential oil of Helichrysum italicum (Roth) G. Don. Determination of ester bonded acids and phenols.* Retrieved from Pubmed: https://www.ncbi.nlm.nih.gov/pubmed/18463581

Meyer JJ1, A. A. (1996). *Inhibition of herpes simplex virus type 1 by aqueous extracts from shoots of Helichrysum aureonitens (Asteraceae).* Retrieved from Pubmed: https://www.ncbi.nlm.nih.gov/pubmed/8733118

Miller, R. A. (1990). *The Magical and Ritual Use of Perfumes.* Destiny Books.

MILLINGEN, J. G. (1839). *Curiosities of Medical Experience ... Second edition. Revised and considerably augmented.* Richard Bentley.

Mojay, G. (1996). *Aromatherapy for Healing the Spirit: Restoring Emotional and Mental Balance with Essential Oils.* Healing Arts Press.

Neville, K. (2016). *The Aromatherapy Garden: Growing Fragrant Plants for Happiness and Well-Being.* Timber Press.

Nostro A, B. G. (2001). *Effects of Helichrysum italicum extract on growth and enzymatic activity of Staphylococcus aureus.* Retrieved from Aromatic Science: http://www.aromaticscience.com/effects-of-helichrysum-italicum-extract-on-growth-and-enzymatic-activity-of-staphylococcus-aureus-3/

Nostro A1, C. M. (2002). *Helichrysum italicum extract interferes with the production of enterotoxins by Staphylococcus aureus.* Retrieved from Pubmed: https://www.ncbi.nlm.nih.gov/pubmed/12180937

Nostro A1, C. M. (2003). *Evaluation of antiherpesvirus-1 and genotoxic activities of Helichrysum italicum extract.* Retrieved from Pubmed: https://www.ncbi.nlm.nih.gov/pubmed/12585233

Nostro A1, C. M. (2004). *Modifications of hydrophobicity, in vitro adherence and cellular aggregation of Streptococcus mutans by Helichrysum italicum extract.* Retrieved from Pubmed: https://www.ncbi.nlm.nih.gov/pubmed/15059215

Ornano L1, V. A. (2015). *Chemical composition and biological activity of the essential oil from Helichrysum microphyllum Cambess. ssp. tyrrhenicum Bacch., Brullo e Giusso growing in La Maddalena Archipelago, Sardinia.* Retrieved from Pubmed: https://www.ncbi.nlm.nih.gov/pubmed/25492232

Oshadhi. (2016, 04). *Helichrysum: Golden Magician of the Sun.* Retrieved from https://oshadhi.life/2016/04/14/helichrysum-golden-magician-of-the-sun/

Padecky, K. (2008, 07). *Essential oil of the Month: Helichrysum*. Retrieved from http://kalasgems.com/Newsletters/helichrysum.pdf

Parkinson, J. (1640). *Theatrum Botanicum: the Theater of Plants. Or, an Herball of a Large Extent* .

Rigano D1, F. C. (2012, 12). *A new acetophenone derivative from flowers of Helichrysum italicum (Roth) Don ssp. italicum*. Retrieved from Pubmed: https://www.ncbi.nlm.nih.gov/pubmed/25285382

Rigano D1, F. C. (2013, 12 12). *Intestinal antispasmodic effects of Helichrysum italicum (Roth) Don ssp. italicum and chemical identification of the active ingredients*. Retrieved from Pubmed: https://www.ncbi.nlm.nih.gov/pubmed/24140587

Robert, A. G. (2005). *The role of aromatherapy in the treatment of viral hepatitis*. Retrieved from International Journal of Aromatherapy: http://www.sciencedirect.com/science/article/pii/S0962456205000640

Rodrigues AM1, S. L. (2015, 08). *Glandular Trichomes and Biological Activities in Helichrysum italicum and H. stoechas, Two Asteraceae Species Growing Wild in Portugal*. Retrieved from Pubmed: https://www.ncbi.nlm.nih.gov/pubmed/26227726

Rose, J. (1993). *The Aromatherapy Book: Applications and Inhalations*. North Atlantic Books.

Sala A, R. M. (2002). *Anti-inflammatory and antioxidant properties of Helichrysum italicum*. Retrieved from Aromatic Science: http://www.aromaticscience.com/anti-inflammatory-and-antioxidant-properties-of-helichrysum-italicum-2/

Sala A1, R. M. (2002, 03). *Anti-inflammatory and antioxidant properties of Helichrysum italicum*. Retrieved from Pubmed: https://www.ncbi.nlm.nih.gov/pubmed/11902802

Sala A1, R. M. (2003, 01 24). *A new dual inhibitor of arachidonate metabolism isolated from Helichrysum italicum*. Retrieved from Pubmed: https://www.ncbi.nlm.nih.gov/pubmed/12559384

Sandal, H. (2014, 09 19). *Helichrysum - Benefits and Uses*. Retrieved from Hosursandal.com: http://www.hosursandal.com/helichrysum-essential-oil/

Schnaubelt, K. (2011). *The Healing Intellegience of Essential Oils,*.

Stewart, W. (1998). *Dictionary of Images and Symbols in Counselling*. Jessica Kingsley Publishers,.

Stillpoint Aromatics. (n.d.). *Helichrysum Italicum Essential Oil Corsica*. Retrieved from Stillpoint Aromatics: http://www.stillpointaromatics.com/helichrysum-italicum-neral-acetate-corsica-essential-oil-aromatherapy

Stupar Miloš (Faculty of Biology, I. o. (2014, 04). *Antifungal activity of Helichrysum italicum (Roth) G. Don (Asteraceae) essential oil against fungi isolated from cultural heritage objects.* Retrieved from Directory of Open Access Journals: https://doaj.org/article/44fa2223591441f1a3092d51adf90670

Sun DX1, L. J. (2011, 11 24). *Reversible inhibition of three important human liver cytochrome p450 enzymes by tiliroside.* Retrieved from Pubmed: https://www.ncbi.nlm.nih.gov/pubmed/21031626

Taglialatela-Scafati O1, P. F. (2013, 03). *Antimicrobial phenolics and unusual glycerides from Helichrysum italicum subsp. microphyllum.* Retrieved from Pubmed: https://www.ncbi.nlm.nih.gov/pubmed/23265253

Teal, C. (2012). *Chiron The Wounded Healer.* Retrieved from Moon Valley Astrologer: http://www.moonvalleyastrologer.com/wp-content/uploads/Chiron.pdf

The Dreaming Earth Botanicals. (2015, 03 03). *http://www.dreamingearth.com/blog/helichrysum-essential-oil/.* Retrieved from The Dreaming Earth Botanicals: http://www.dreamingearth.com/blog/helichrysum-essential-oil/

The Rose and The Amaranth. (n.d.). Retrieved from Sacred Texts: http://www.sacred-texts.com/cla/aesop/aes312.htm

Tundis R, S. G. (2005). *Influence of environmental factors on composition of volatile constituents and biological activity of Helichrysum italicum (Roth) Don (Asteraceae).* Retrieved from Aromatic Science: http://www.aromaticscience.com/influence-of-environmental-factors-on-composition-of-volatile-constituents-and-biological-activity-of-helichrysum-italicum-roth-don-asteraceae/

Tyler, G. (2013, 03 07). *HElichrysum/everlasting/Immortelle essential oil.* Retrieved from Homeopathy Gina Tyler: https://homeopathtyler.wordpress.com/2013/03/07/helichrysumeverlastingimmortelle-essential-oil/

Valkyrie Astrology. (n.d.). *Chiron The Wounded Healer.* Retrieved from http://www.valkyrieastrology.com/Makeover/asteroids/chiron.html

Vesta Lyn. (n.d.). *Chron in The Houses.* Retrieved from https://vestalyn.wordpress.com/2014/03/07/chiron-in-the-houses/

Walker, S. (2015, 03 09). *Come, see a helichrysum hydrosol distillation.* Retrieved from https://khlorisbotanical.com/helichrysum-hydrosol-distillation/

Walt, L. V. (2005, December). *Helichrysum splendidum.* Retrieved from Kirstenbosch National Botanical Garden: http://www.plantzafrica.com/planthij/helichrysumsplend.htm

Worwood, V. A. (n.d.). *The Fragrant Heavens.* Random House Books.

Wreford, J. T. (n.d.). *Working with Spirit: Experiencing <i>Izangoma</i> Healing in Contemporary South Africa.*

Young, R. T. (2013). *Essential Oil Safety: A Guide for Health Care Professionals.* Elsever Helath Sciences.

Zane Stein. (2012). *Chiron and Friends.* Retrieved from http://www.zanestein.com/ChironCalculator.htm

Zeljković SĆ1, Š. M. (2015). *Volatiles of Helichrysum italicum (Roth) G. Don from Croatia.* Retrieved from Pubmed: https://www.ncbi.nlm.nih.gov/pubmed/25675145

Disclaimer
by SEQ Legal

(1) Introduction

This disclaimer governs the use of this book. [By using this book, you accept this disclaimer in full. / We will ask you to agree to this disclaimer before you can access the book.]

(2) Credit

This disclaimer was created using an SEQ Legal template.

(3) No advice

The book contains information about aromatherapy and the use of essential oils. The information is not advice, and should not be treated as such.

[You must not rely on the information in the book as an alternative to qualified medical advice from a health professional. advice from an appropriately qualified professional. If you have any specific questions about any medical matter you should consult an appropriately qualified professional.]

[If you think you may be suffering from any medical condition you should seek immediate medical attention. You should never delay seeking medical advice, disregard medical advice, or discontinue medical treatment because of information in the book.]

(4) No representations or warranties

To the maximum extent permitted by applicable law and subject to section 6 below, we exclude all representations, warranties, undertakings and guarantees relating to the book.

Without prejudice to the generality of the foregoing paragraph, we do not represent, warrant, undertake or guarantee:

that the information in the book is correct, accurate, complete or non-misleading;

that the use of the guidance in the book will lead to any particular outcome or result; or in particular, that by using the guidance in the book you will heal disease or work in any way as a cure for illness.

(5) Limitations and exclusions of liability

The limitations and exclusions of liability set out in this section and elsewhere in this disclaimer: are subject to section 6 below; and govern all liabilities arising under the disclaimer or in relation to the book, including liabilities arising in contract, in tort (including negligence) and for breach of statutory duty.

We will not be liable to you in respect of any losses arising out of any event or events beyond our reasonable control.

We will not be liable to you in respect of any business losses, including without limitation loss of or damage to profits, income, revenue, use, production, anticipated savings, business, contracts, commercial opportunities or goodwill.

We will not be liable to you in respect of any loss or corruption of any data, database or software.

We will not be liable to you in respect of any special, indirect or consequential loss or damage.

(6) Exceptions

Nothing in this disclaimer shall: limit or exclude our liability for death or personal injury resulting from negligence; limit or exclude our liability for fraud or fraudulent misrepresentation; limit any of our liabilities in any way that is not permitted under applicable law; or exclude any of our liabilities that may not be excluded under applicable law.

(7) Severability

If a section of this disclaimer is determined by any court or other competent authority to be unlawful and/or unenforceable, the other sections of this disclaimer continue in effect.

If any unlawful and/or unenforceable section would be lawful or enforceable if part of it were deleted, that part will be deemed to be deleted, and the rest of the section will continue in effect.

(8) Law and jurisdiction

This disclaimer will be governed by and construed in accordance with English law, and any disputes relating to this disclaimer will be subject to the exclusive jurisdiction of the courts of England and Wales.

(9) Our details

In this disclaimer, "we" means (and "us" and "our" refer to) [Build Your Own Reality)] of [Sy8 1LQ].

Recipes

Skin Repair After Operation

Helichrysum x 1

Myrrh x 1

Camomile matricaria x 1

50 ml (2 fl oz) Rosehip oil

Apply three times a day. Add to the wound dressing if necessary.

Blood Thinning

Helichrysum x 1

Holy Basil x 1

Spikenard x 1

In 50ml (2fl oz) Borage Oil

Safety- Not recommended until after 16 weeks of pregnancy

Reduction of Cholesterol

Helichrysum x 1

Grapefruit x 1

Rosemary x 1

In 50ml (2fl oz) Borage Oil

Safety- Not recommended until after 16 weeks of pregnancy

Heart Protection

Rose x 2

Geranium x 3

Helichrysum x 1

Use in an aromapendant to calm the stress and send healing molecules to the brain, but also the lungs to distribute in the blood stream

Liver Protection

Carrot x 2

Rosemary x 1

Helichrysum x 1

In 50ml (2fl oz) Borage Oil

Safety- Not recommended until after 16 weeks of pregnancy

Apply three times daily to the outside of the right leg, rubbing up and down to activate the liver meridian.

Gall Bladder

Helichrysum x 1

Peppermint x 2

Bergamot (FCF) x 2

In 50ml (2fl oz) Tamanu Oil

Safety- Not recommended until after 16 weeks of pregnancy. Do not use after 6 pm at night so the peppermint does not affect sleep.

Apply three times daily to the outside of the right leg, rubbing up and down to activate the liver meridian which works in tandem with the gall bladder.

Pancreas

Holy Basil x 1

Helichrysum x 1

Lemon x 1

In 50ml (2fl oz) Pumpkin Seed Oil

Safety- Not recommended until after 16 weeks of pregnancy

Apply three times daily to the abdomen and lower back.

Anti-Inflammatory

Yarrow x 2

Helichrysum x 1

Camomile Matricaria x 1

In 50ml (2fl oz) Blank Ointment

Safety- Not recommended until after 16 weeks of pregnancy

Apply as often as is required by the pain.

Chirotic Abscesses

Helichrysum x 1

Galbanum x 1

Geranium x 1

10ml (2fl oz) Calendula Carrier Oil

Mix into 40 ml (1 ¾ oz) Blank Ointment.

Apply three times a day for a month.

Stretch Marks

Centella asiatica x 2

Helichrysum x 1

Frankincense x 2

25 ml (1 fl oz) each of Rosehip and hibiscus oils

Digestive

I made this blend with ginger from *Sanatio Naturalis* and myrrh from *Boswellness* as a recipe for a man's handcream. The artisan distilled myrrh and the unusually deep ginger note were exquisite. Seek them out. You won't be disappointed I assure you. It is sexy beyond belief.

Ginger x 1

Helichrysum x 1

Myrrh x 1

In 50ml (2fl oz) Pumpkin Seed Oil

Safety- Not recommended during pregnancy

Apply three times daily to the abdomen and lower back.

Coughs and Chest congestion

Helichrysum x 1

Benzoin x 1

Monarda x 1

In 50ml (2fl oz) Blank Moisturiser

Safety- Not recommended until after 16 weeks of pregnancy

Apply three times daily to the chest and back

Anti-Aging Moisturiser

Neroli x 1

Helichrysum x 1

Frankincense x 2

5ml Wheat Germ Oil

In 50ml (2fl oz) Blank Moisturiser

Safety- Not recommended until after 16 weeks of pregnancy

Toner

Helichrysum Hydrolat

Carrot x 5

Petitgrain x 5

25 ml (1fl oz) Witch hazel

Acne treatment

Helichrysum x 2

Jasmine x 1

Lavender x 1

Vetiver x 1

In 50ml (2fl oz) Blank moisturiser

Safety- Not recommended during pregnancy

Metaphysical

I have not included carriers or methods of use because these can only really seen in the context of the patient and what they are able to use. Perhaps they will want bath oils, massage oils diffuser. Only you as the therapist can construe what will work best. These mixes are purely suggestions and you will be able to create your own based on the problems you find before you.

1st House Issues to do with self-worth

Basil, Thyme, Helichrysum

2nd House to do with money and fixations on possessions

Ginger, Helichrysum, Bergamot

3rd House Problems with learning

Melissa, Clary Sage, Vetiver, Helichrysum

4th House needing to be needed

Jasmine, Helichrysum, Myrrh

5th House Sat of the Moment

Basil, Helichrysum, Jasmine

6th Feelings of incompleteness

Helichrysum, Vetiver, Clary sage

7th Relationships

Helichrysum, Rose, Palma Rosa

8th House Birth and Death

Spikenard, Helichrysum, Rose

9th House – Feelings of intellectual inferiority

Helichrysum, Geranium, Cedarwood

10th House - Problems setting Goals

Helichrysum, Bergamot, Spikenard

11th House- Friendships

Ylang Ylang, Cypress, Helichrysum

12th House - At Odds with oneself

Black Pepper, Rosemary, Helichrysum

www.ingramcontent.com/pod-product-compliance
Ingram Content Group UK Ltd.
Pitfield, Milton Keynes, MK11 3LW, UK
UKHW020142250726
13967UKWH00002B/822